Dr Marios Kyriazis is an internationally acclaimed pioneer in the science and application of anti-ageing medicine. He is a practising physician who has also studied gerontology (the science of ageing) at King's College, University of London. He has a Diploma in Geriatric Medicine from the Royal College of Physicians of London and he is a Chartered Biologist and member of the Institute of Biology for work into the biology of ageing.

He is the founder of The British Longevity Society and is an advisor to several other age-related organisations. He has published over 400 articles on healthy ageing, both for scientists and for the public.

By the same author

The *Anti-Ageing* Plan

Stay Young Longer — Naturally

The Look Young Bible

CARNOSINE

And Other Elixirs of Youth

The Miraculous Anti-Ageing Supplement

Marios Kyriazis MD

Watkins Publishing
London

This edition published in the UK in 2003 by
Watkins Publishing, 20 Bloomsbury Street, London, WC1B 3QA

NOTE FROM THE PUBLISHER
Any information given in *Carnosine and Other Elixirs of Youth* is not intended to
be taken as a replacement for medical advice. Any person with a condition
requiring medical attention should consult a qualified medical practitioner
or suitable therapist.

Cover design by Echelon Design
Cover photograph © GettyOne
Designed and typeset by Jerry Goldie and WestKey
Printed and bound in Great Britain by NFF Production

British Library Cataloging in Publication data available

Library of Congress Cataloging in Publication data available

ISBN 1 84293 049 4

www.watkinspublishing.com

Contents

To Stella

Acknowledgements

I would like to express my thanks to the following who helped in one way or another:

Professor Alexander Boldyrev of the Lomonosov Moscow State University, for support and advice; Dr Mark Babizhayev for providing details about the ophthalmic uses of carnosine; Dr Alan Hipkiss, of the University of London, for useful discussions; Dr Jay Olshansky, of the University of Illinois, for criticising some of the issues surrounding anti-ageing treatments; International Anti-Aging Systems for providing the carnosine and for initiating dialogue.

Introduction

We live in the era of information. Until a few years ago, people who had no medical knowledge were happy just to follow the advice of their doctor, without asking too many questions. Nowadays there is so much medical and health-related information available to the general public, that any intelligent person is eager to try and learn more about how to maintain their own health. People are not satisfied with blindly accepting medical advice, and they want to cross-reference, check and expand on their knowledge of their medical condition.

Health matters such as the ageing process are not considered quackery any longer, and have little to do with monkey glands and snakeskin elixirs, but are legitimate areas of scientific research. Interest in this area is increasing by the day and new supplements and drugs are being made available to the general public, sometimes bypassing the need to consult with a doctor. This creates the potential for misinformation or self-treatment with the wrong medication. This book aims to dispel any clouds of misinformation, while educating intelligent people who want to take an active part in managing their own health.

I started working in the field of anti-ageing medicine over fifteen years ago, when I could see that medical advances would inevitably help every one of us live longer than our parents and grandparents. I was also aware that medical information would be made available to a much larger section of the public and this would create the necessity for science-oriented doctors to scrutinize the amount of sound, reliable information reaching the public, and to filter out nonsensical concepts and quack medicine.

In those days carnosine was an ideal supplement to concentrate on because it appeared to be a multi-purpose, easy to obtain, natural anti-ageing agent. My interest in carnosine developed over the past twelve years as more research results were being made available, confirming my initial feelings about its effectiveness.

This book offers you the chance to learn something about the intricacies of the ageing process, and to get some 'inside' information on how ageing can affect you. I will start by explaining some of the simple concepts, and then tackle in earnest some of the dark and difficult to understand aspects of ageing. My aims are simple and practical. The first is to discuss and explain the actions of the nutrient carnosine and to highlight the importance of using it. My second aim is, by explaining the many puzzling details of the ageing process, to provide you with enough knowledge to enable you, with the help of your physician, to choose your medication in an informed, rather than a haphazard, fashion.

Before I discuss the benefits of carnosine, we need to explore in some detail the basics of the ageing process. I do not assume that you have any previous knowledge of the subject, but I will gradually go into it in sufficient depth to stimulate the interest even of those with a relatively advanced understanding of ageing. Let me start by answering a few questions people may have about ageing.

What is Ageing?

The prestigious scientific journal, *Biogerontology*, defines ageing as: 'The progressive failing ability of the body's own intrinsic and genetic powers to defend, maintain and repair itself in order to keep on working efficiently'.

Traditional scientists believe ageing to be a natural phenomenon which is:

- intrinsic (in our genes)
- deleterious (detrimental with no benefits)
- universal (affecting every living thing)
- progressive (going only in one direction and irreversible).

Cutting-edge thinking however, shows that this view is becoming difficult to support. Although ageing is indeed written into our genes, it is not completely irreversible. The clock has been turned back in a number of pioneering experiments during the past few years and, on at least one occasion involving ground-breaking cloning techniques, it has been reset to zero.

Ageing is certainly not due to a simple lack of a hormone or nutrient. Taking supplements or replacing a single nutrient is not going to reverse ageing. It is a much more complicated process than that, and there are several different mechanisms involved in it. Some of these mechanisms overlap, others are independent, but all of them are complicated. Any book trying to explain ageing for lay people is bound to be simplistic so, if you do find the following discussion difficult, bear in mind that in real life things are even more complex than this.

Is Ageing a Disease?

The simple answer is 'no'. Contrary to what many people – including some doctors and scientists – believe, ageing is not a disease.

Consider the following common condition – someone who, because of their age, is unable to talk properly, too weak to walk and confined to bed, with a severely reduced sense of balance, unable to feed themselves and relying on the care of others, they are incontinent of urine and faeces, and have a very poor memory. Is this person ill? Of course not, I am talking about a baby here. This baby may or may not have an illness which affects babies, such as nappy (diaper) rash or abdominal colic, but it is not ill merely because it has the characteristics of a baby.

It is the same with ageing. Ageing as such is not a disease, but just another period in our normal life. There are diseases which can affect anybody but which are, in fact, more common in later life – such as strokes and heart disease, diabetes, certain types of cancers, dementia, osteoporosis and arthritis. Young children can also have arthritis or cancer, teenagers can have diabetes, and twenty-year-olds can die of a heart attack. These are illnesses, and should not be confused with the natural underlying process of ageing. Ageing is a natural phenomenon and it is a progressive inability of the body to maintain and repair itself. Fighting age-related illness is one thing, fighting the ageing process is another. Having said that, however, many natural ageing mechanisms frequently result in actual diseases, so fighting an ageing process may well bring about an improvement of an age-related illness.

Ageing has been a fact of life since life was first created. All animals or plants, even if they are protected from an early death caused by predators or disease, will eventually show signs of ageing. Many people use chemicals extracted from plants to help them ward off the signs of ageing. Have you ever wondered why we have this natural inclination to choose plant chemicals in our fight against illness? Nature created these plant chemicals with the sole aim of protecting plants against disease or ageing. Humans came along afterwards and adapted these chemicals for their own use, to increase their chances of maintaining their health.

Humans have always been able to live for many years and also to experience at least some of the signs of ageing. During certain periods of human evolution, ageing was only experienced by very few people, and then only a small minority of those people lived to a very old age. Nowadays, many more people live to reach 'old age' (75–80 years) and even more live to a 'very old age' (90–100 years). The average lifespan is, as we know, increasing.

Surprisingly, there are still respectable scientists out there who believe that the average human lifespan cannot increase any more. They believe that it would be impossible for most people to live to the age of 85 or more. I remember how in the 1970s scientists were claiming that the average lifespan simply could not be extended beyond 80 years of age. Now that this limit is being reached, these scientists have changed their position and increased their estimate to 85 years of age. In a few years they will probably change their minds again and increase the limit to 90. In fact, there are other equally respectable scientists who claim that, with time and effort, it will be possible to extend the average human lifespan to around 110–120 years: that is to reach the maximum limit of a natural lifespan.

Beyond that age, the estimates and speculation enter the realms of science fiction, and so I am not going to discuss this further. People who claim that we will be able to live to an age of 200 and beyond, are simply looking too far into the future in a way that is not relevant to us, our children or our grandchildren. Perhaps genetic science will make the steps that are necessary to achieve that unnatural age, but this is not going to happen in our time or during the next generation.

What is Anti-Ageing Medicine?

Anti-ageing medicine is a branch of medical science and applied medicine, aimed at treating the underlying causes of ageing and at alleviating any age-related ailment, with the ultimate goal of extending the healthy lifespan of humans. It aims not only to prevent and reduce the severity of age-related diseases – arthritis, dementia, cataracts for example – but also to prevent and reduce the severity of ailments which are due to the natural process of ageing, such as skin ageing, and the loss of muscle tissue, and so maintain some of the characteristics of youth.

It uses conventional and alternative regimes in an integrated approach to achieve the best possible result for the patient. It is a holistic discipline, seeing the patient as a whole and not just as an isolated disease. Perhaps one of the most important characteristics of anti-ageing medicine is that it is not so much concerned with treating existing diseases, but rather with preventing future age-related health problems.

Many people claim to be experts in anti-ageing medicine, when in fact they have not had any suitable training. Some are not even medical practitioners. Others use the term 'anti-ageing medicine' rather liberally to include quack treatments and therapies which have no scientific basis whatsoever. Interested individuals can study age-related medicine at accredited universities, and there are also other courses of study, for example those offered by the American

Academy of Anti-Aging Medicine, which is, however, not formally accredited by the medical profession.

Anti-ageing medicine is not merely geriatric medicine. Geriatric medicine is the treatment of old people who are ill, whereas anti-ageing medicine is aimed at both young and old people who want to prevent age-related problems for as long as possible, and to maintain health into old age. According to one of the first modern anti-ageing physicians, the Romanian Professor Ana Aslan, treating ageing is both 'a science and an art'.

Some scientists and doctors are uncomfortable with the term 'anti-ageing medicine', because they think it is unscientific. They suggest more scientific-sounding, pompous terms such as 'interventive biogerontology' or even 'strategies for engineered negligible senescence (SENSe)'. The latter term basically means to artificially slow down ageing to almost zero. These terms may have relevance in scientific circles but they do not change the general meaning of what anti-ageing medicine is. My grandmother used to say, 'John is still John, no matter how he dresses.' You can change the terminology as much as you like, but the underlying essence of anti-ageing medicine will remain the same.

What is Youth?

Youth, in the context of anti-ageing medicine, is taken to mean not merely not being old, but possessing some, or all, of the characteristics of idealized youth, for example:

- good health
- strong muscles
- an efficient immune system
- a sharp memory and a healthy brain
- hormones working at their peak capacity

It does not matter how old you actually are: in other words, it is not a matter of chronological age, but a matter of improving a person's biological, social, spiritual and mental state. Somebody is considered 'aged' or 'old' who has succumbed to the problems related to age. You may be of an advanced chronological age but still retain some of the characteristics of youth. For example, there are 90-year-olds who look healthy, are without any significant illnesses, feel energetic and enjoy life to the full. They are content and fulfilled, and enjoy the best of both worlds – the health of youth plus the wisdom of age.

Anti-ageing medicine is not necessarily directed against all ageing as such, but only against the medical or health problems of ageing. Some aspects of ageing can be really beneficial. For example, wisdom and understanding of the world increase with age, spiritual matters are better appreciated, and there are even some physical areas which improve with age:

- allergies generally become less troublesome
- travel sickness is less likely to occur
- sensitivity to pain decreases.

By the same token, youth is not necessarily a totally good thing, and certain aspects of it – such as health and a youthful appearance – are more desirable than others. Inexperience and insecurity, for example, are definitely seen as undesirable in the eyes of many older people. Youth should not be confused with a young chronological age. What most people are trying to achieve is not a young chronological age but a young biological age – they want to be healthy and biologically efficient.

What is an Elixir of Youth?

An elixir, disregarding the mythical, alchemical and unscientific connotations, is a solution or mixture of chemicals used as a medicine or for treatment. There is a subtle difference between 'the elixir of life' (a preparation which is intended to prolong life indefinitely) and the 'elixir of youth' (a preparation which can maintain youth as defined above). In this book I am not talking about prolonging life indefinitely but about prolonging some of the characteristics of youth.

Words

A lot of people, including some respectable scientists, are in a muddle about the different terms used in the anti-ageing field. They use words like 'longevity', 'immortality' and 'rejuvenation' without making a distinction between them. These words may sound as if they refer to similar things but there is, in fact, a great difference between them. Any linguist will tell you that 'longevity' simply means 'long life'. An anti-ageing physician will tell you that longevity does not mean merely prolonging life for the sake of it, but also extending the number of years you can live in good health. Those who are opposed to pursuing longevity, thinking that its aim is merely to add years to life, irrespective of all the illnesses that come with that, are simply mistaken. 'Longevity', in the eyes of an anti-ageing practitioner, is not one, but two things – living longer and being healthier.

You will notice that when I speak of 'living longer' I am not specific and do not refer to any numbers. How much longer? Longer than what? The answers are vague. By as much as possible. Longer than others. I think by 'a long life' most people mean an age of 90–95 years, whereas a minority may mean an age of over 100.

Other terms used in the anti-ageing field are:

- 'rejuvenation' which means 'to make young again'
- 'eternal life' means living forever. 'Forever' can, however, mean different things for different people. Some take it to mean 200–300 years of age, whereas others consider it to mean 1000 years. Some people take it literally, really forever.
- 'immortality' means never dying, which is, in a sense, similar to the above terms.

Notice that none of the above terms says anything about being healthy or unhealthy. They should be used correctly and not too literally. Treatment with a certain product will not make you 'immortal', but may grant you a certain degree of 'longevity'. Future treatment with genetic manipulation may bring about 'rejuvenation' but not 'eternal life'.

Animal Experiments

In this book I refer extensively to research done not only on cells in the laboratory but also to experiments performed on animals such as rats, mice, dogs, and rabbits. If you are seriously against animal experimentation then you will need to decide whether this book is for you or not. Whether I oppose or support animal experiments is not a relevant issue here. I am merely reporting on what other people have already done. My own experiments are based solely on consenting human volunteers, who are fully informed about their treatment.

There is an important distinction to be made between results based on animal studies and those based on studies with humans. The majority of the results presented in this book are based on animal studies. Although there are certain biological similarities between animal and humans, this does not mean that a positive result from an animal study will necessarily hold true for humans as well. Many, if not all, manufacturers of anti-ageing products quote positive research results but they do not always make a distinction between animal and human research.

In many situations, animal research can help us to better understand ourselves, and lays the foundations for human experiments. Quite often the human studies happen to agree with results from animal studies but this is by no means always the case. So I would warn you against being taken in by enthusiastic advertisements, which claim positive findings unless these have been shown to be true specifically for humans.

Any type of scientific research, even research published in established, prestigious journals, can easily be criticized and flaws can be found. At university we were given classic excerpts from scientific articles (such as those describing the discovery of DNA) and asked to find flaws in them, as an exercise. We were always successful. People who are opposed to anti-ageing medicine may criticize some of the studies mentioned in this book. This is nothing unusual, it is an established scientific practice. The studies are presented as a whole, to give a sense of the general direction of the research and are not to be taken in isolation or at face value.

There is a difference between an 'experiment' and a 'clinical trial'. An experiment is when a treatment or a procedure is tried on animals or humans in artificial and controlled surroundings. A clinical trial is when a drug treatment is given to human patients, in real situations, who are then monitored to see what happens to them. For the sake of simplicity, I use these two terms without making a distinction.

Pioneering Treatments

All of the treatments referred to in this book form part of anti-ageing medicine, which is a new and pioneering medical discipline. By definition, pioneering means that we are not sure what is over the horizon. It is inevitable that there will be a degree of speculation and conjecture as well as uncertainties, contradictions and uncorroborated evidence regarding the treatments. Anti-ageing medicine is still not a fully established discipline, and if you decide to use its treatments you should understand that nothing is guaranteed, at least not in the sense of traditional, established medical disciplines. You should be willing to be flexible, tolerant, open-minded and curious to find out more about a particular drug.

An important point is that, whereas research may not yet fully support the use of a product, this product may actually work for you as an individual. On the other hand, research may support the use of a product which happens not to be particularly effective for you. So it is a matter of personal experimentation, trial and error, based on what current science has to offer.

Using Anti-Ageing Drugs or Supplements

I take it as a given that people who want to use any of the supplements or drugs referred to in this book, will only do so under medical or expert supervision. Some of the drugs mentioned are only available on a doctor's prescription, but others are not. There is no point in taking anti-ageing medicines without a clearly defined personalized plan which takes into account your own particular requirements, any illnesses or medical conditions, other drugs you may be taking, your lifestyle and any other relevant factors. The dose of each of these medicines needs to be adjusted depending on the individual, and only a specialist practitioner will have the necessary expertise to create a personalized plan for you. Taking anti-ageing medicines without expert supervision is not only a waste of money but you must be aware that it could also be dangerous.

Many general practitioners and family physicians have developed an interest in non-conventional treatments and are very well placed to give background medical advice regarding the supplements mentioned in this book. However, this may not be true for every family doctor, so if you think that your questions remain unanswered it may be worth consulting a specialist anti-ageing health practitioner such as a nutritionist, a gerontologist or an anti-ageing physician. Information on how to locate a suitable practitioner near you may be available from some of the organisations listed at the end of the book. They should be able to help you choose which supplements to take, if any, and monitor any possible benefits and side effects.

Chapter 1

Ageing and What Causes It

There are several theories about what causes ageing. Some of these contradict each other, whereas some others overlap. Some make logical sense, whereas others do not. During a recent anti-ageing conference, we were ten people on a panel, drawn from a wide variety of scientific backgrounds, to answer questions from the audience. Towards the end of the session, one participant asked each one of us the simple question, 'What causes ageing?' The answer was not simple. In fact, there were ten almost completely different answers.

For the purpose of understanding ageing and making better sense of the treatments available I am going to concentrate on only a small number of the relevant theories. These not only make some sense but have an important plus – they give you the chance of doing something practical about your own ageing. These theories do not depend on some scientist using genetic engineering to extend the lifespan of fruit flies or worms, they do not depend on a high-tech company researching gene manipulation, and they are not about dull scientists churning out theoretical and academic jargon. The theories are based on practical, down-to-earth concepts which can easily be adapted and employed by anybody, in an attempt to enjoy a healthy life for as long as possible.

There are three main biochemical processes involved in ageing. These are oxidation, glycosylation and methylation. Other processes which can also have practical relevance are those involved in chronic inflammation or hormonal dereg-ulation. The following is a very simple introduction to the biology of ageing, examining these processes.

Oxidation

Most people have heard about the mayhem free radicals cause to your body. Free radicals are a group of simple compounds with an electron missing from their chemical structure and this makes them unstable. They seek out other chemical structures from which they can acquire an electron.

Free radicals are like single men at a married ladies' party. A single man at such a party would not just sit quietly looking out of the window, but would try to find a partner from the abundance of women available. When that single man did find a partner, it would mean that the husband of that woman would be without a wife, he would be angry and would go on to cause trouble, quite understandably. The party would end in disaster. This is exactly what happens when a free radical reacts with your tissues, causing a lot of heavy and permanent damage, leaving your body as devastated as a party which ended in a serious fight.

To be fair, free radicals in small and controlled quantities are useful in your everyday metabolism. They take part in several normal reactions within the body and they help you to breathe and consequently to live. The majority of free radicals are produced during oxygen metabolism, within your cells. When production of these free radicals increases and goes out of control, then the problems start.

One old proverb says that you are better able to fight your enemies if you give them a name. So here are the names of some free radicals:

- superoxide radicals
- hydrogen peroxide
- hydroxyl radicals
- nitric oxide

The scientific names for some of the different types of free radicals are reactive oxygen species (ROS, or oxygen free radicals), reactive nitrogen species (RNS, or nitrogen free radicals) and so on.

The human body has developed several effective ways of dealing with these troublemakers. Examples of these methods of defence are:

- the inactivation of a free radical within the cell just after its creation
- the mopping-up of free radicals by scavenging antioxidants

3

● the increased elimination of material already
damaged by free radicals

Returning to the party analogy, trouble would be prevented if
the single man was not there in the first place, and similarly
we can avoid exposure to free radicals from such sources as
pollution, bad diet, and smoking. His being stopped at the
door could be likened to free radical inactivation and if he was
picked up inside the room by a wandering bouncer we could
compare that with free radical scavenging. If, as soon as he
finds his woman, he is escorted out of the party immediately
we have the analogy with the elimination of already damaged
material. So, you see that there are several stages which lead to
complete free radical mayhem, but potential problems can be
prevented at each one of these different levels.

Examples of some of the antioxidants, or free radical
fighters, in your body are the vitamins A, C, E, the mineral
selenium, and such chemicals as catalase, superoxide
dismutase (SOD) and glutathione. But there are hundreds
of others.

One part of the cell which is most susceptible to free radical damage is its outside shell, i.e. the cell membrane. The cell
membrane is composed mainly of lipids (fat) and proteins.
The lipids on the membrane are very liable to interact with
free radicals and produce a chemical called malondialdehyde
(MDA) which we will be referring to later on in the book. MDA
is a dangerous by-product of free radical activity and can
cause further harm to your tissues. There are many other
by-products of free radical damage, which not only cause

further damage themselves, but also contribute to another important ageing process called glycosylation which I will discuss a little further on.

What You Can Do to Reduce Free Radical Injury

Oxidation is the price you pay for breathing oxygen. Oxidation creates free radicals which contribute to ageing. You can limit your exposure to free radicals in a variety of ways: I have already mentioned avoiding smoking, pollution and a bad diet, all of which can increase the production of free radicals and deplete your body of antioxidants. Everyone knows the benefits of a healthy, active lifestyle and I do not need to discuss these here.

Another way of limiting free radical hits is to take more antioxidants, both in the diet and by supplementation. There are people who say that it is not necessary to use supplements, and that humans have managed to survive for thousands of years without taking antioxidant tablets. The problem is, however, that we now live in a technological era which, for the first time in human history, increases our exposure to free radicals through artificial radiation, the depletion of the ozone layer, pollution with chemicals in every part of the 'civilized' world, stress, hormone-treated animals and toxins in foods. Under these circumstances, it is not unreasonable to assume that you might need to supplement your intake of dietary antioxidants with additional supplements in tablet form, in order to counteract all the hostile aspects of our modern environment.

Examples of common antioxidants, apart from those which I have already mentioned are:

- pycnogenol
- lutein
- co-enzyme Q10
- isoflavones in general

These and many others are found in plant chemicals (phytochemicals) as well as in fish and animal products. Consuming a diet rich in fruit, dark-coloured vegetables, fish and lean meat can go some way to providing your body with certain necessary antioxidants, but you also need to take supplements for the reasons I have already given. I will be discussing two of these supplements, carnosine and Q10, in more depth later on in the book. Some of the natural antioxidants not only fight free radicals but can also take part in other processes such as glycosylation. Carnosine is a typical example of an antioxidant which is also an anti-glycosylation nutrient.

Glycosylation

Before I move on to another age-related process, that of glycosylation, let me briefly explain what a protein is. Proteins are valuable biological molecules which play a huge part in maintaining normal life. They are found in almost every part of the body and have a variety of functions. For example, proteins are present inside the cells, carrying oxygen and other nutrients to the tissues and making the life of the cell possible. They are also present outside the cell as parts of the immune system fighting bacteria and viruses.

Proteins are formed by long strings of amino acids. These are relatively simple chemicals – lysine, methionine, and arginine, to mention a few. If you imagine a protein as a wall, amino acids are the individual bricks. However, proteins are not straight lines of amino acid sequences, but have a certain normal configuration.

For example, in a three-dimensional world, a particular protein may go five amino acids straight up, six amino acids to the left and down, three towards you, five to the right and up, and so on, making it a complex structure like a very twisted stick. Any change to this configuration and the protein loses its normal function. You will see why this normal protein configuration is so relevant when I discuss glycosylation.

The process of glycosylation (also called glycation) is turning out to be almost as important as oxidation in causing age-related damage. Glycosylation happens when glucose molecules (and other sugars such as fructose, or other similar chemicals such as aldehydes) attach themselves to proteins. MDA (malondialdehyde) is an aldehyde which is very keen to take part in this reaction. Other aldehydes which can also take part in glycosylation are acetaldehyde and the more familiar formaldehyde.

This attachment of sugars to proteins is responsible for causing a brownish discoloration of tissues. This is not as innocent as it might sound. Why? Because this combination of sugars and proteins (i.e. glycosylation) causes proteins to bind to each other. Let me explain why this matters.

Normally, proteins are not supposed to be bound to one another. There are exceptions, of course, but let us concentrate for a moment on this rule:

- protein does not, and should not attach to another protein
- protein can attach to sugar
- sugar can attach to protein

Therefore, the end result of this is that a protein, which is attached to a sugar is liable to interact with, and bind to, another protein. This is called 'cross-linking' and is not good news at all.

Imagine your hands are two individual proteins. They are free to do what they like, when they like, independent of each other. They are there to serve you and protect you. Move them around. They are not bound together. Bring your thumbs together and try to keep them attached to each other. Nothing happens. Your hands are still free to move around. Now imagine putting a good amount of extra strong glue – the equivalent of a sugar molecule – on one thumb – the equivalent of a part of the protein. Bring your thumbs together again. You will see that your thumbs now bind firmly together, making your hands unable to move independently and unable to do anything useful. This is 'cross-linking' in all its glory.

A cross-linked protein is not only useless but can cause more damage by reacting with free radicals and other toxins to create grotesque biological material called advanced glygosylation end-products (AGEs). These are the equivalent of what happens when your thumbs are cross-linked, i.e. when they are glued and bound together. You will start dropping things on the floor, spilling your drink, making a mess, all of which makes life more difficult.

Just as with the free radicals and the party analogy mentioned above, there are several intermediary stages during the process of glycosylation. These stages, with their 'thumb' analogies are:

Stage 1. The approach of a sugar/aldehyde molecule to the protein − getting the glue ready

Stage 2. The actual attachment of the sugar/aldehyde molecule to the protein and the creation of an activated protein, ready to be cross-linked − applying glue on the thumb. This particular step is called 'carbonylation', see below.

Stage 3. The cross-linking of the proteins − the binding together of the two thumbs

Stage 4. The formation of AGEs − the combination of the two disabled thumbs and the damage they cause as a result.

Also, as with the free radicals and the party analogy, there are different steps where glycosylation can be blocked. Referring to the above four stages, here is a possible plan of action:

Protection step 1. Avoid exposure to glycosylating agents – by avoiding a high carbohydrate diet – or block these as soon as they are formed – inactivate MDA for example

Protection step 2. Immediately cover or protect the carbonylated protein – for example, by using carnosine, as will be explained below

Protection step 3. Break the bond between these proteins, or get rid of those proteins which are already cross-linked

Protection step 4. Fight AGEs and related damage with antioxidants and with other anti-ageing drugs.

The reason why AGEs are called 'advanced' glycosylation end products, is simply because they are the end result of an advanced stage of the glycosylation process (stage 4). These monstrosities are real troublemakers, circulating in the body and causing a lot of harm, contributing heavily to what we call 'ageing'. AGEs cause further cell damage when they attach themselves to the cells, at special attachment sites called RAGEs (receptors for AGEs). When they bind to the cells they stimulate the production of several poisonous chemicals within the cell. The end result is destruction of the cell, plus creation of further toxic by-products (MDA for example) which start all over again in a vicious circle.

AGEs are found in most tissues of your body, and increase constantly from the age of twenty onwards. A large amount of AGEs in the brain has been blamed for contributing to Alzheimer's dementia, because AGEs increase the formation of beta amyloid. This is a toxic material found in the brains of older people and it is particularly abundant in Alzheimer's dementia patients. Apart from beta amyloid, AGEs also stimulate the production of other dangerous compounds such as certain free radicals (including nitric oxide or NO) and others such as interleukin-6 and tumour necrosis factor. I will explain more about these toxic, inflammatory compounds later on.

Let me return to the details of cross-linking. I have explained how 'bad' chemicals such as aldehydes and sugar derivatives, can bind to proteins and 'turn them bad'. This particular step in the process of glycosylation (stage 2 in the above example) is so important that it has its own name. It is called 'carbonylation'. This means that the sugar compounds add chemicals called 'carbonyl groups' to the protein in preparation for a full cross-linking.

Ageing is associated with an increased number of carbonyl groups on proteins which is a way of saying that during life many of our proteins get earmarked for destruction and can do little else but get cross-linked. About a third of all human proteins become carbonylated in later life. A carbonylated protein is like a thumb with glue on it, ready to be cross-linked at any moment.

I mention all of these apparently complicated steps for a reason. As you will see later in chapters 2 and 3, cutting-edge research shows that the nutrient carnosine can block these carbonylated proteins and inactivate them, preventing them from being cross-linked. Returning to the analogy of the glue on your thumb, if you stick a piece of paper on your glued thumb before you touch the other thumb, then your thumbs may look a mess but they will not attach to each other, leaving you free to move your hands. Here, carnosine is the equivalent of the piece of paper. A protein which has been protected by carnosine is said to be 'carnosinylated'. This is a protective benefit of carnosine which tries to patch up carbonylated proteins before they attach to other proteins.

So, to summarize:

- A protein with a carbonyl group on it is called 'carbonylated' — glue on thumb.
- A carbonylated protein which has reacted with carnosine is called 'carnosinylated' — piece of paper on the thumb with the glue.
- A carbonylated protein which does not have the benefit of carnosine protection and has been allowed to react with another protein is called 'cross-linked' — two thumbs glued together.

As mentioned above, MDA is a real troublemaker — the equivalent of the glue — attaching itself to healthy proteins and making them liable to be cross-linked. Where does it come from? It is the result of free radical damage to lipids (fatty constituents of cells). You see now how oxidation and glycosylation are linked. Oxidation creates free radicals which produce MDA which causes glycosylation which results in AGEs which create more free radicals which produce MDA which . . . and so on, until you die.

However, all is not lost. There is hope, in the guise of the nutrient carnosine. It can break this cycle because it interferes with MDA. It does this in the following ways:

A. It combines with MDA and inactivates it before it can cause any damage (the equivalent of prevention step 1 above). This is how lipofuscin is formed. Lipofuscin is a relatively inert material found in increased amounts in your tissues during ageing, manifesting as brown skin spots for example. Lipofuscin is a sign that a reaction has already taken place, either a reaction between MDA and protein which is bad, or MDA and carnosine which is good, because it means less MDA. There are two kinds of lipofuscin: the one formed by carnosine and MDA is harmless, whereas that formed by protein and MDA may be harmful.

B. It repairs proteins already damaged by MDA, those carbonylated proteins which, although not cross-linked yet, are ready to be cross-linked in a short time (the equivalent of prevention step 2 above). The carbonyl group is covered and inactivated by carnosine so the protein cannot cause any more harm through being cross-linked. These proteins are then eliminated in several stages and taken out of the system (part of prevention step 3 above).

Ordinary antioxidants such as vitamins E and C are active against free radicals but they do not do anything against glycosylation. Carnosine, however, is active both against free radicals and against glycosylation. One reason why carnosine is effective against glycosylation is because its chemical structure is similar to that of other chemicals which cause glycosylation, and it can therefore easily attach itself onto the protein, protecting it against any intruders.

Examples of clinical impairment resulting from glycosylation are:

- The wall of the arteries becomes thick and inflexible and crumbles easily, resulting in high blood pressure, heart attack or stroke.
- The inside of the brain cells gets clogged with abnormal biological material (beta amyloid) resulting in loss of memory and contributing to dementia.
- The skin proteins and collagen clump together, and then collapse to form wrinkles and grooves on the skin.

Unfortunately, the process of glycosylation not only affects proteins but also interferes with the DNA. For example, sugar molecules can cause abnormal bonding between a DNA molecule and a protein, also called cross-linking. A cross-linked DNA molecule is of no use at all. The trouble with glycosylation was always thought to be that the bonds it forms are permanent. When two proteins (or a protein and a DNA molecule) are cross-linked, it was forever. We can prevent cross-linking but we could not break the abnormal bonds formed between two already cross-linked molecules.

This is very important because it illustrated the irreversibility of ageing. When the damage had already been done we could do nothing to reverse it. If we were able not only to prevent, but also to reverse cross-linking, if we could break the bonds already formed between two proteins, then in effect we would be reversing ageing, making the proteins 'young' again (the equivalent of prevention step 3 above).

Until now, breaking existing bonds between already cross-linked proteins *was* thought to be impossible. Not any more. Later on I will discuss further a new, state-of-the-art group of drugs (for example, one called ALT711) which can actually break existing bonds between proteins, which is the equivalent of applying special solvent to two glued thumbs, dissolving the bond and freeing the hands again. This shows that ageing is not completely irreversible. Let me now move on to another important age-related process, that of methylation.

Methylation

During methylation, chemicals called 'methyl groups' are being added to different constituents of the proteins, DNA and other molecules to keep them in good, active condition. Examples of useful chemicals which need to be methylated are:

- the antidepressant, 'feel-good' brain chemical, serotonin
- the useful stimulant hormone, adrenaline
- the 'good' fat molecules, HDL
- certain constituents of the cell membrane called phospholipids (including the chemical phospha-tidyl-choline).

Without methylation, none of the above chemicals would be able to stay around for long. Generally speaking, methylation is necessary for the normal maintenance of your tissues, and it is usually kept at healthy levels naturally by your body. However, like most processes related to ageing, things are not that simple. While moderate methylation is good, excessive and unbalanced methylation is not something you would want. I will explain why, shortly.

A good aspect of methylation is that methyl groups move around the blood stream, piggybacking on special chemicals. These carrier chemicals are called 'methyl donors' because they donate their extra methyl groups to any other molecules that need to be methylated. One of these methyl donors is called SAMe (S-Adenosyl-Methionine) which is one of the most important methylators in the body. Another methyl donor is TMG (tri-methyl-glycine), which, as the name suggests, carries three methyl groups. It is a kind of molecular camel, laden with its cargo of methyl groups. I will refer more to these two friendly compounds in chapter 7.

A few examples of situations where methylation is essential are:

1. A methylation process transforms the nutrient carnosine into its cousin called 'anserine' which is a more stable and not so easily destroyed compound.
2. Methylation of certain parts of your DNA causes the permanent switching off of unnecessary genes and saves your body from abnormal DNA division. This means that methylation of those particular sections of DNA

blocks any abnormal DNA from being passed on to future generations of cells.

3. Methylation of the dangerous chemical homocysteine transforms it into the harmless amino acid methionine.

4. The amino acid arginine needs to be methylated to its sister molecule called 'mono-methyl-arginine' which is a really useful compound to have in the brain. It adjusts certain brain receptors (binding sites), particularly the NMDA receptor which plays a part in inflammation and excitotoxicity, two age-related processes, which will be briefly discussed later in the book.

The problem is that methylation can plummet during certain stages of life. For example, any chronic inflammation process can affect methylation because the immune system, which is heavily involved in fighting inflammation, gorges itself on methyl groups, leaving nothing for other tissues of the body. From this example you can see the overlap of two theories of ageing, the theory of methylation and that of inflammation. One process can affect the other, and fighting one aspect of ageing may have a repercussion on other parts.

Low methylation is reflected in the increasing levels of the nasty chemical homocysteine, which is found in chronic inflammation processes such as lupus, heart disease and diabetes. An increased intake of methylators has been shown to reduce the risk of these diseases. Heavy exercise also increases the demand for methylating chemicals to fuel the muscles during exercise, so methylation for the rest of the body takes second place, and becomes neglected. The moral of this? Do not exercise excessively.

Unbalanced Methylation

The bad news is that methylation is not completely foolproof. Yes, it is useful for some body parts, but if left unbalanced, it can deregulate other parts. It can, for example, switch off useful genes which protect you against cancer, or it can activate other genes which promote cancer. The methylation process becomes relatively unbalanced during ageing, resulting in DNA, collagen and protein destruction, as well as interfering with several normal reactions which are thirsty for methyl groups.

Everything involved in ageing is a matter of balance. Too much is bad. Too little is also bad. Some methylation is essential, and any age-related loss of methylation increases the rate of cell death. Free radicals add insult to injury in this respect by speeding up the destruction already caused by defective methylation. On the other hand, certain parts of the DNA, if excessively methylated, may also cause damage or even cancer.

Are there any practical steps you can take to help yourself? Your body is usually a good judge regarding which parts need methylating and which parts do not. So if you try to keep a good level of methylating nutrients in your diet and take methylating supplements, (see chapter 7) your body will then decide how best to use these for its own benefit.

Other Processes Involved in Ageing

Apart from the trio of oxidation, glycosylation and methylation, there are two other main processes which are implicated in nature's devilish plot to age you. One is chronic inflammation and the other is hormonal deregulation. Let us deal with inflammation first.

There are scientists who believe that most age-related changes in the body are due to chronic inflammation. When there is chronic inflammation the body tissues are eaten away by toxic chemicals, resulting in dementia, thickening of the arteries, arthritis, diabetes, hormonal imbalance and so on.

A particular component of chronic inflammation is excitotoxicity. This happens when the brain cells are overexcited. The brain chemical, glutamate, is normally responsible for stimulating the different parts of the brain, but too much glutamate results in overexcitation and the eventual death of the cell. The results of excitotoxicity are seen in strokes and Alzheimer's dementia. As I shall explain, carnosine protects against excessive glutamate activity, and thus reduces excitotoxicity.

The chemical MDA has also been implicated in inflammation – as if its behaviour in causing glycosylation was not enough – and so carnosine, which hates MDA, has anti-inflammatory benefits. Chronic inflammation has been associated with a chemical called tumour necrosis factor

19

(TNF) which is found to be high in Alzheimer's disease and in multiple sclerosis, to give two examples. TNF actively promotes degeneration of your brain and nerves. It is activated by a combination of AGEs and free radicals, so carnosine plays a useful role in preventing this.

Chronic inflammation and brain damage can also be caused by a dangerous by-product of nitric oxide (NO), called peroxynitrite. This is the result of the oxidation of NO, and it is a major toxic by-product. It can, for example, worsen atherosclerosis. Antioxidants (such as co-enzyme Q10) may help foil the actions of peroxynitrite.

A handful of doctors suggest that people should be using low doses of anti-inflammatory chemicals such as aspirin, ibuprofen or diclofenac to keep age-related inflammation at bay. This is not a widely shared opinion however. A diet containing nutrients which can reduce some of the effects of inflammation is, however, a good idea. Such a diet should include fish (which contains anti-inflammatory oils), fruit and vegetables (particularly berries which are packed full of antioxidants and inflammation-fighting flavonoids) and supplements of alpha lipoic acid which is a well-known inflammation fighter.

Hormones

Now we come to the fifth and final major process involved in ageing, and that is hormonal deregulation. This theory says that ageing results in a general hormonal imbalance within the body. In plain terms, your hormones go haywire with the passage of time.

Drs Dillman and Dean explained the effects of this hormonal imbalance, and if you are interested in exploring this further, you need to read their book *The Neuroendocrine Theory of Ageing and Degenerative Disease* (The Center for Biogerontology, Pensacola, Florida 1992). What has relevance here is that hormones such as growth hormone, melatonin and DHEA need to be replaced or reactivated during ageing to prevent your body from falling apart. Not only that, but the binding sites, where the hormones attach themselves onto the cells need to be in good working order, otherwise the hormones will be unable to operate properly.

Some scientists, however, flash a warning. Your supplies of growth hormone or DHEA may well dry up as you grow older, but perhaps this reduction is not a dangerous thing after all, and may happen for a reason. It may, for example, prepare your body to become better able to cope with the changes of increasing age. Those who gorge themselves on extra supplements of hormones may be interfering with a natural defensive mechanism, throwing a spanner in the normal workings of hormonal balance. Some scientists even say that growth hormone replacement may accelerate ageing, in the long term.

This is one point of view. Many anti-ageing doctors, though, believe the opposite is true. They believe that if the level of something is high in youth and low in old age, then replacing that something should make the physical aspects of youth reappear.

So, these are the main processes of ageing and I trust that this discussion of them opens up some opportunities for action which may protect you against the devastation ageing can cause. Many people ask me whether ageing can be reversed. My answer is that it depends on what you mean by 'ageing'. Commonly available products cannot reverse all aspects of ageing as a whole. They may be effective on a single age-related process such as oxidation, glycosylation, methylation, or inflammation, but they are not able to influence the entire ageing process. Anti-ageing medicine uses products or procedures which claim to be able to:

A. *Protect* against ageing and here this is taken to mean 'certain parts of ageing' such as oxidation, glycosylation, or inflammation. The products used include carnosine, co-enzyme Q10 and antioxidants, which may attack only one or two of the mechanisms of ageing.

B. *Reverse* a. the 'signs' of ageing through the use of DHEA, growth hormone, face lifts and skin products, for example. These can change the way you look but they do not affect your rate of biological ageing.
b. actual biological ageing through the use of ALT711, telomerase or cloning. Such methods have been shown actually to reverse biological ageing and turn back the clock in a limited way, on a handful of occasions.

You will see from what I have said that the 'elixirs of youth' I discuss have good points and bad points. Some of them are not so well studied, whereas others are studied but with negative results. Only carnosine has consistently produced positive results, in study after study. So without further ado, let us look closely at carnosine.

Chapter **2**

A Basic Introduction to Carnosine

I magine it is the year 1900. In a cold Russian laboratory two scientists by the names of Gulewitsch (also spelled Gulevitch) and Amiradzibi, slowly add different chemicals to pots of mashed muscle tissue. Amiradzibi stirs the test tubes, boiling them and adding alcohol to the concoction, while Gulewitsch checks the results and, every now and then, scribbles down some unreadable series of complicated chemical formulas.

Suddenly one of them stops and looks with amazement at his test tube. For a few minutes only the rain falling on the dirty windows of the institute breaks the uncanny silence. But the quiet is soon shattered by the researchers' excited conversation. The two scientists now check their results again and again not believing their very eyes. A hitherto unknown compound is lying at the bottom of one of the test tubes. Carnosine has been discovered!

Their results are eventually published in a German magazine under the title *'Uber der Carnosin, eine neue organische Base des*

Fleischextrakten' – which translates as: '*On Carnosine, a new organic base extracted from flesh (muscle)*'. And then comes the anticlimax. Scientists at that time were more concerned about mapping the different parts of the cells, and so a publication about a simple muscle extract did not attract much attention. Their article, covering just two short pages of the magazine, was soon forgotten.

Over the years, scientists have realized that carnosine is not just a small insignificant molecule but that it has a surprising range of health benefits. The majority of the research has been performed in Russia behind closed doors, inaccessible to the West. Carnosine remained forgotten by almost every Western researcher, languishing in scientific oblivion for decades. It is only in recent years, since the collapse of the former Soviet Union that the Russian researchers' findings have reached the eyes of Western scientists. When they realized what carnosine had to offer, some of these Westerners were so excited that they changed their entire careers, dedicating their lives to the study of carnosine.

I remember about ten years ago, one of these scientists told me, in confidence, that the benefits of a secret chemical he was studying were so far-reaching that he could not tell me the name of the actual substance. He called it 'substance X', in the spirit of a true Russian spy. Actually Dr Alan Hipkiss of the University of London was not Russian at all, but British, and his secret 'substance X' was, in fact, carnosine.

Although several British, Australian and Japanese, but surprisingly few Americans are now researching carnosine full-time, it is the Russians who produce the majority of the research papers on it. One of them, the famous researcher Professor Alexander Boldyrev of the Moscow State University, has studied carnosine extensively and has been instrumental in helping us understand its benefits. During my correspondence with him it became obvious that he is one of the most knowledgeable scientists about carnosine in the world today. Together with Hipkiss and a handful of others he tells us everything there is to know about carnosine.

What is Carnosine?

Carnosine is the result of the marriage between the amino acids b-alanine and L-histidine. Not surprisingly its chemical name is 'b-alanyl-L-histidine'. The facilitator of this union bears the unromantic name of 'carnosine-synthetase'. This is an enzyme which, as the name suggests, synthesizes carnosine from its individual constituents.

Some people confuse carnosine with another chemical called 'carnitine'. This, however, has nothing to do with carnosine and it just happens that these two have similar-sounding names. The same is true for other variants of these two compounds. For example, I will refer later to acetyl-carnosine which has nothing to do with acetyl-carnitine.

Carnosine is found in massive quantities in muscle, including the heart muscle, where it is one of the most abundant chemical compounds, and in the brain, particularly in the olfactory nerve, which is responsible for the sense of smell. Smaller quantities are also present in the kidneys and in the stomach.

It is no coincidence that carnosine is mainly found in tissues that live relatively longer than other tissues of the body. Muscle and brain cells usually live longer than say, red blood cells, skin cells or bowel-lining cells. This may be significant because it says something about the potential properties of carnosine. Cells that die quickly are replaced equally quickly. It does not matter if they get damaged by ageing, because they will soon be replaced by new and healthy ones. However, cells that live for a long time – such as muscle and brain cells – once they are injured they may not be replaced and we are stuck with them. These damaged cells are useless for our survival. Therefore, something has to be done to protect them in the first place, before they get irreparably harmed.

For this reason, nature has taken extraordinary steps to protect long-lived tissues, and has deployed one of its most effective weapons – carnosine. Usually, under natural conditions, biological compounds have many different functions. Carnosine is a glaring example of this rule, as we shall see later on.

Sources of Carnosine

Some animal or fish species (such as carp) do not contain any carnosine, whereas others are brimming with it. Examples of carnosine-rich tissues are:

- chicken breast
- rabbit leg
- frog
- sturgeon
- beef leg
- duck and turkey meat

In birds, carnosine is much more concentrated in the breast than in the thighs. This is perhaps due to the fact that breast muscles are much more useful during flight than thigh muscles, and nature is therefore protecting the valuable breast muscles with a valuable chemical. It may please men to know that the concentration of carnosine is higher in their muscles than in those of women, probably for the same biological reasoning as above – because men are supposed to be stronger and to run faster than women, so they require extra protection for their muscles.

The overall concentration of carnosine in both animal and human tissues dwindles with age. For example, in some instances, the carnosine levels may plummet by 10% every 10 years. This lack of carnosine may be due to the loss of muscle tissue which is a common legacy of increasing age. Less muscle tissue means less carnosine.

Muscular Power

From experiments performed several years ago it was concluded that giving extra supplements of carnosine in tablet, eye-drop or injection form, did not increase the concentration of carnosine in the tissues, but that this extra

Some Interesting Facts about Carnosine

- In ducks carnosine appears for the first time 17 days prior to hatching.
- Dolphin muscle contains more carnosine than cat muscle.
- Oysters, squid and octopus do not contain any carnosine at all, although they are rich in alanine, which is one of the constituents of carnosine.
- In certain birds, carnosine is converted into its cousin anserine, as soon as the birds acquire the ability to fly.

carnosine was either eliminated in the urine or inactivated by special enzymes. This was disappointing news initially, but thankfully more recent experiments have shown this not to be entirely the case. Japanese scientists have found that giving rats extra carnosine in the diet can indeed increase the concentration of carnosine in rat muscles. In these experiments, a very high intake of carnosine resulted in a fivefold increase of the carnosine concentration in muscle.

As far back as 1953 scientists realized that adding a spoonful of carnosine to a quantity of tired muscle tissue in the laboratory could reverse fatigue and enable the muscle to work at full power again. This effect was given the name 'Severin's phenomenon' after its discoverer, Dr S. Severin, and it is one of the reasons why Russian and other athletes continue to take carnosine supplements for improving endurance and muscle function before an important athletic event.

There is limited research which suggests that, for some reason as yet unknown, endurance training may actually suppress natural carnosine concentration in the muscle. If this is true, then taking extra supplements of carnosine may help your body to perform better during periods of physical training. One explanation for the loss of carnosine is that excessive and prolonged exercise fuels the production of those silent but deadly free radicals which speed up ageing. Because carnosine is an antioxidant, it is soaked up quickly during the body's effort to fight these free radicals. The message here is that too much exercise is not a good idea at all, because it accelerates ageing. It is best to exercise moderately, perhaps for only 30 minutes at a time.

There are several similar variants of carnosine, and the following are examples:

- anserine (produced by methylation of carnosine)
- homocarnosine
- N-acetyl-carnosine (also called N-alpha-acetyl-carnosine)
- carcinine

There is a formidable array of at least 29 other variants of the carnosine family. These are called 'imidazole di-peptides', for the very simple reason that they are groups of two amino acids (hence di-peptides) containing the chemical structure 'imidazole' as their backbone. Most of these have benefits similar to those of carnosine proper.

Is Carnosinase a Good or a Bad Terminator?

Once created, a molecule of carnosine cannot just stay around for ever, as it is soon inactivated by an enzyme called carnosinase. This is a sort of terminator which has only one aim in life – to destroy the bond connecting the two individual amino acids forming carnosine, and so to release alanine and histidine. Incidentally, in biology anything ending in '-ase' usually means 'an enzyme that interferes with other substances'.

When carnosine is injected into the muscle, it can reach the body tissues quickly but it is then tracked down and attacked within an hour by carnosinase. On the other hand, experiments show that after taking carnosine supplements by mouth, a relatively large amount (14%) can be found in the urine even five or six hours afterwards. This means that carnosine given by mouth has the ability to pass through the intestine and navigate through the blood to reach the tissues, whereas carnosine by injection is quickly inactivated by carnosinase and eventually lost.

The concentration of the enzyme carnosinase corresponds to the actual levels of carnosine in the tissues: the higher the amount of carnosine, the higher the concentration of carnosinase. The brain, for example, contains significantly higher amounts of carnosinase. It is as if carnosinase homes in to carnosine whenever it sees it and wrestles it to the ground.

Carnosinase comes in different variants, which are found in the blood (serum), kidney and brain as already mentioned. Other less important variants can be found in the liver. Carnosinase is not always very efficient actually inside the cell and so as soon as carnosine manages to leave the blood and enter the cell it is relatively safe.

I have explained that carnosinase breaks carnosine down to its individual constituents, histidine and alanine. Carnosine is one of the least toxic compounds so there is no apparent reason why nature would have gone to the trouble of creating carnosinase to inactivate this non-toxic nutrient. There must be another reason for the presence of carnosinase. While some people believe that carnosinase is harmful, because it destroys carnosine, others are not so sure. The breaking down of carnosine to histidine and alanine may be a valuable natural source of these two amino acids.

Alanine, for example, is needed during processes which stimulate the formation of new genetic material and new collagen, whereas histidine fights muscle fatigue and stabilizes the inflammation reactions following an allergy. It can also reduce the severity of breathing difficulties experienced by some athletes after strenuous exertion.

It turns out however, that carnosine's benefits are not entirely due to just alanine and histidine, because when these two nutrients are given separately, they do not always work as well as carnosine does. In experiments with mice, for example, carnosine can make the animals look younger in appearance, but any treatment with alanine plus histidine

– given as two individual compounds – has no effect at all. Strange but true!

In any case, carnosinase also has an appetite for other variants of carnosine albeit to a lesser extent. For example, carnosinase is four times less potent against anserine, and it has almost no effect on N-acetyl-carnosine. This shows that a small chemical modification of the structure of carnosine can result in a much stronger and virtually indestructible product, well protected against carnosinase.

Let me tell you about an ancient Greek general called Kimon who was so fearsome that, even before a battle, his enemies fled in terror. He was once getting ready to attack a mighty Persian army but he caught the flu and died. His successors decided to continue with the campaign without spreading the news of his death. Sure enough, they confronted the Persians who, fearing the great general Kimon, surrendered without a fight. So, the motto of Kimon from then on was 'Kai Necros Enika' which means 'Even when he was dead, he was victorious'. In some way, as I explain below, this motto should perfectly fit carnosine.

Carnosine is a fearsome compound as it is, but when it is broken down by carnosinase and 'dies', its benefits do not cease. It releases alanine and histidine which are then used for the formation of other much needed chemicals such as those which form part of the DNA. So, in a way, carnosine, even when it is dead, is still effective and enables us to win our fight against ageing.

The individual components of carnosine – alanine and histidine – need to be examined in some more detail.

ALANINE

Alanine on its own (i.e. when it is not incorporated onto the carnosine structure) is an important amino acid found in muscle tissue. It is obtained from beef and pork, oats and wheatgerm, and cheese, yoghurt and other dairy products.

Sometimes alanine supplements are used by diabetics who want to reduce the high amount of sugar in their blood. Alanine can also stimulate certain special immune cells, the leukocytes, and can therefore benefit people who have a weak immunity.

It is present in the prostatic fluid, (the fluid produced by the prostate to lubricate the sperm) and some men are now using alanine to boost the health of their prostate. At least one scientific study has revealed that taking alanine supplements can limit the symptoms of benign prostatic enlargement. No side effects or interactions have been reported.

HISTIDINE

If you consume enough meat, poultry, fish, wheat, rice and rye, you should be getting sufficient supplies of histidine. This amino acid is invaluable during normal growth and repair. It preserves the protective myelin sheath around the nerves, flushes out toxic metals from the body and balances the stomach fluids. People with rheumatoid arthritis frequently have reduced reserves of histidine, and so they take extra histidine supplements for its possible benefits.

Many histidine users report improved sexual arousal and better enjoyment of sex. High amounts of histidine in the diet increase the levels of carnosine itself in the tissues. Histidine-related compounds, including carnosine, are generally good antioxidants and regulate the normal death and replacement of cells, which brings me directly to the process of apoptosis.

Normally, your cells wither and die in an orderly and controlled manner, during a natural process called 'apoptosis'. It is necessary for cells to die when they become damaged beyond repair, to give a chance to new healthy cells to grow and replace the old and worn out ones. Apoptosis is a programmed cell death, a kind of weeding-out of weedy cells. A slow, constant rate of apoptosis is normal, but a speeded up rate is excessive and results in the loss of a large number of cells. For this reason, apoptosis needs to be regulated and allowed to tick over at a slow rate. Histidine, carnosine and similar compounds do exactly this: they regulate apoptosis and so suppress any excessive loss of cells.

Wheezing, Sneezing and Itching

When carnosine is broken down by carnosinase, the process releases histidine which is then liable to be chemically transformed into another compound called histamine. This is an old foe which most people are familiar with. Too much of this stuff can cause allergic reactions such as: hay fever, skin rash, asthma, or even shock. That is where the anti-histamine drugs come in, to block this excessive production of histamine and thus reduce allergic reactions.

I have spoken to several patients and to some doctors who are worried about the potential of carnosine to be transformed into histamine. Their rationale is that, because histamine causes allergies, carnosine — which may turn into histidine, and eventually into histamine — also has the potential to cause allergies, so its use should be restricted.

As with most physiological processes, moderation and balance are the key words. An excessive amount of histamine can go out of control and can indeed cause allergic reactions, but a small, well-controlled amount of histamine is necessary for the normal day-to-day management of your body. Histamine is created during times of stress and it is then used to keep stress under control. It can, for example, regulate the blood flow to the kidneys, which helps flush out toxins produced during stress.

Given that small amounts of histamine are necessary to protect you during stress, carnosine which, under certain circumstances, can be transformed into histamine, can be really useful here. It immediately supplies that extra histamine which is necessary so that the body can go about its everyday routine uninterrupted. Carnosine, far from causing histamine toxicity, turns out to be a useful agent which can reduce some of the effects of stress.

Surprisingly, carnosine does not cause allergies. On the contrary, it is an allergy-fighter which can block or reduce skin allergies. I have explained how under normal circumstances, a small amount of carnosine is turned into the histamine necessary for our usual, day-to-day needs. When too much histamine is produced, carnosine immediately comes to the rescue. It blocks the histamine receptors on the cells and so leaves the histamine molecules stranded and helpless. If histamine is prevented from binding to the cells it becomes unable to cause any allergies or toxicity.

So, although carnosine has the theoretical potential to produce too much histamine which may result in allergies and shock, actually the opposite happens. Carnosine modulates and balances the actions of histamine. As I have said when too much histamine is in circulation, carnosine blocks it and when too little histamine is around, carnosine produces extra supplies, to help top up and maintain a healthy level.

This example illustrates the complexity of the different biological mechanisms. Things appear deceptively simple, but they are surprisingly complicated. Only by understanding the way a particular substance works, will you be able to use it to your benefit.

A Really Hard Worker

Anybody reading about carnosine will be immediately struck by the extraordinary range of its actions. It has three full-time functions, and several part-time ones. Its main functions are:

- a buffer/chelator of toxic substances
- an antioxidant
- a natural anti-glycosylator.

CARNOSINE AS A BUFFER/CHELATOR

Let me explain briefly what 'chelator' means. A chelator is a chemical which engulfs metal ions, smothers them and inactivates them. Chelators work more or less like buffers, substances which bind to any toxic chemicals inside the cell and disarm them. Carnosine has the posh scientific title of 'intracellular buffering agent and heavy metal chelator'.

Let us say you go out for your daily jog. You manage to go a certain distance and then you notice that your leg muscles start to ache. What causes this aching? The answer is simple. During exercise, your muscles generate lactic acid as a by-product of the energy used by the exercising muscle. Increased quantities of lactic acid cause the familiar muscle pain. It is now time for carnosine to go to work. Together with its cousin, anserine, it can cushion the impact which lactic acid has on the muscle cells, and so it restores the normal equilibrium within the cell. Carnosine acts as a chemical buffer reducing lactic acid in your muscles. This particular action of carnosine, however, is much more pronounced in sprinting animals, and only of limited importance in humans.

Muscle groups which need a huge amount of energy and create a lot of fast movements (breast muscles, in birds, body muscles in fish, leg muscles in frogs, rabbits and other sprinting animals), are very rich in carnosine. One reason for this is that nature needs carnosine to be where a large amount of toxic chemicals are generated, so that it will inactivate them quickly. Because of this buffering ability, carnosine is useful in preventing and reversing muscle fatigue. This is the basis of the Severin phenomenon, discussed earlier. Carnosine also helps maximize respiration, induce healthy sleep and decrease blood pressure by relaxing the muscles within the blood vessel wall.

Inside the cell, carnosine chelates (binds to, and inactivates) metal ions such as:

- copper
- zinc
- aluminium
- vanadium
- cobalt, and other heavy metals.

Copper and zinc are needed during the normal workings of the nerve cells, but excessive zinc or copper activity can be toxic and contribute to stroke, dementia or epilepsy. Carnosine regulates the concentration of these and many other metals. If the metals are abnormally low, carnosine increases their concentration. If they are dangerously high, it lowers them.

Carnosine goes a bit further than merely binding to the metal and inactivating it. Importantly, the resulting carnosine–metal combination is not biological junk at all but a useful chemical in itself! For example, carnosine–copper compounds are good antioxidants, whereas carnosine–zinc compounds are effective anti-ulcer agents. Carnosine takes a bad thing (excessive copper or zinc metals) and does not just neutralize it, but turns it into a positively handy chemical. That's clever! This property of carnosine may turn out to have useful applications in diseases in which there is a degree of copper or zinc toxicity, and so it may protect against dementia, stroke and fits.

Zinc which is bound to carnosine forms a chemical called 'zinc-carnosine chelate compound' or just 'Z-103'. This is an effective treatment for ulcers, protecting the lining of the stomach against free radical attack. Zinc on its own or carnosine on its own do not have any appreciable benefits on the lining of the stomach, but the combination of the two is superb. Not only does the Z-103 compound heal existing ulcers, but it can also prevent further ulcers from being formed.

In an experiment, this preventative bonus of the Z-103 compound was found to be relatively similar to that of the prescription drug cimetidine. One of the reasons for this could be the histamine-blocking ability of carnosine, as explained above. Too much histamine binds to certain stomach cell receptors called H2 and floods the stomach with hydrochloric acid which may result in ulcers. Both Z-103 and cimetidine block this H2 histamine receptor preventing the histamine from causing damage.

I will deal with this further in the next chapter, where I discuss another carnosine–zinc drug with the trade name of Polaprezinc. As well as carnosine–zinc compounds, other carnosine–metal compounds are deadly against stomach ulcers. As far back as 1982, experiments showed that carnosine–aluminium compounds protected against stomach ulcers in rats, whereas carnosine or aluminium given separately did not have any effects on the ulcers.

Some people use a chemical called EDTA – in tablet form or by injection – which is an effective metal chelator, just like carnosine. EDTA binds to heavy metals and eliminates them. This, on the face of it, appears to be a sensible drug to use. However, experiments also show that when there are no heavy metals around, carnosine cannot function to its full extent. For example, the combined efforts of carnosine and heavy metals help glucose molecules stay out of your tissues. Remember that too much glucose lingering in your tissues accelerates glycosylation and this worsens ageing.

Carnosine–metal combinations reduce glucose by stimulating its transformation into valuable energy. But, when there are no heavy metals around – for example when somebody has already removed them with EDTA – then carnosine remains stranded and can do nothing much on its own. As you can see it could be better to let carnosine, rather than EDTA, bind to and inactivate heavy metals. This is because the compounds resulting from the binding of carnosine to heavy metals are very useful for other reactions down the line, whereas the combination of EDTA with metal is just neutral and inactive, causing neither harm nor good.

CARNOSINE AS AN ANTIOXIDANT

Another main function of carnosine is to prevent free radical injury, particularly to the fatty components of the cell membrane. Carnosine is a cell membrane stabilizer and protector. Cells with a damaged outside membrane are like balloons with holes in them – useless. Carnosine not only protects the membrane surrounding the cell but also shields the membrane surrounding the mitochondria.

The fatty components of the membrane, particularly those of the mitochondrial membrane, are keen to interact

Mitochondria

- These are tiny organs present inside every cell and are responsible for producing energy from different chemicals.
- The mitochondria are surrounded by their own membrane, so they are like 'cells within cells'. There are over one thousand mitochondria in each cell.
- An intact mitochondrial membrane is vital during energy production.
- Both the cell membrane and the mitochondrial membrane are made up to a great extent from fatty material, such as polyunsaturated fatty acids, which are prone to free radical attack.
- Carnosine and anserine can boost the production of energy within the mitochondria because they facilitate the process of oxidative phosphorylation, an essential energy producing mechanism.

with free radicals during a process called lipid peroxidation. The resulting by-products of lipid peroxidation – one of which is our old friend MDA – end up causing all sorts of further mayhem such as:

- a meltdown of energy production
- an increase of water seepage inside the cells or inside the mitochondria, and
- eventual death of the cell.

All is not lost however. Carnosine can protect against all of these gloomy scenarios. One way it is able to do that is by lending a hand to other antioxidants such as vitamin E and SOD (superoxide dismutase). The benefits are clearly seen when a mixture of several antioxidant vitamins is used. Carnosine is especially fond of vitamin E and works exceptionally well with it. The presence of the one increases the efficiency of the other. This is because carnosine works better in water, whereas vitamin E works in fat, so both watery and fatty tissues are reached.

In experiments with muscle extracts, scientists found that the higher the dose of carnosine, the less damage was caused by free radicals. If used at a certain high level, carnosine is able to stop free radical activity completely. These antioxidant benefits of carnosine are more evident in nervous tissue.

While carnosine helps other antioxidants, it also has anti-oxidant properties itself. It tries to foil any free radical-related crime. Variants of carnosine may or may not be strong antioxidants depending on their chemical structure.

This highlights the fact that the properties of a particular substance depend on many factors and should not be taken for granted.

Carnosine is a reasonably effective free radical scavenger, in that it patrols your tissues and, as soon as it encounters a free radical, binds with it and eliminates it. Specifically, carnosine is effective against a type of free radical called singlet oxygen. However, some scientists believe that carnosine on its own may not be very effective against certain more powerful free radicals, and this is one of the reasons why I recommend the use of other antioxidants in association with carnosine. The triple action of carnosine, co-enzyme Q10 and vitamin E is lethal in the fight against free radicals.

Radiation Hazard

Radiotherapy in the treatment of cancer creates a large amount of free radicals which cripple both the cancer cells and healthy cells alike. Scientists have explored the possibility that carnosine can protect healthy tissues which have been exposed to radiotherapy.

Experiments with mice show that taking high doses of carnosine increases the lifespan of mice which have been exposed to strong radiation. Treatment with carnosine before or during radiation is effective, whereas treatment after the radiation has already been given has no benefits.

CARNOSINE AS AN ANTI-GLYCOSYLATOR

The third full-time function of carnosine is fighting glyco-sylation. As I have explained in chapter 1, glycosylation is the process of forming damaging bonds between proteins and sugars. The result could be the creation of cross-linked proteins and AGEs but carnosine reacts with the carbonyl groups of the proteins, making them less liable to be cross-linked.

Carnosine is powerful in fighting all the stages of glyco-sylation. It is particularly keen at binding to the sites of proteins where sugar/ aldehydes attach. When these sites are blocked, the sugar is unable to react with the protein, and so the protein remains unharmed. Carnosine also locates and protects the chemical deoxyribose (normally found on the DNA molecule) which is a terrifying 200 times more potent at causing glycosylation than glucose is.

This brings us to another potential role of carnosine, the protection of the DNA molecule against glycosylation and eventual cross-linking. In addition, carnosine can help the cell get rid of any abnormal strands of already damaged DNA molecule, leaving the place clear for healthy DNA to multiply.

Brain Power

Now let us look at some of carnosine's part-time activities which you will appreciate better if I just concentrate on the brain. You will see that it can function as a neuro-transmitter – a chemical that helps a message jump from one nerve cell to another – a dementia-fighter, and a memory-boosting nutrient.

The levels of carnosine are very high near the synaptic spaces of olfactory nerve cells. The synaptic space is where one nerve touches another, and where an electrical signal passes from one nerve cell to another. This has made scientists think that carnosine could be a sort of neurotransmitter, particularly in the olfactory nerve, which is responsible for the sense of smell. It is interesting to note that some of my patients, who were completely unaware of this action, reported without any prompting an improved sense of smell after using carnosine for two to three months.

I have already mentioned the metal binding and chelating properties of carnosine, and particularly the benefits of carnosine–zinc or carnosine–copper compounds. The action of carnosine in regulating these two metal ions goes much deeper than simple binding. Let me explain. Small amounts of zinc and copper are found in many parts of the brain but they are especially concentrated in the olfactory nerve, sustaining an acute sense of smell. However, excessive or unregulated amounts of zinc and copper have been linked to over-stimulation of the nerves, causing excitotoxicity, which has been implicated in Alzheimer's, stroke and ageing in general.

For example, zinc or copper stimulates the production of beta amyloid which is a toxic by-product of the brain metabolism, found in the brain of patients with Alzheimer's disease. Beta amyloid is a formidable poisonous material which:

- speeds up the process of apoptosis, (the orderly death of damaged cells), and results in so much apoptosis that very few healthy brain cells remain behind
- worsens the destruction caused by free radicals
- inhibits the normal growth of cells
- is toxic to the blood vessels in the brain.

Carnosine takes part in protecting against beta amyloid-induced injury by binding to the zinc or copper metals and modulating their activity on the nerve receptors. Other chemicals such as aminoguanidine, SOD and glutathione were tested in this respect but it was shown that carnosine works better than all of them.

Some scientists believe that Alzheimer's dementia starts in the olfactory nerve, because the first microscopic changes of dementia are seen in its cells. As a result, the first thing Alzheimer's disease patients notice could be a disturbance in their sense of smell. Because carnosine protects against zinc or copper-related injury it may have an overall protective effect against Alzheimer's.

Apart from this possible defence against Alzheimer's, carnosine plays a role in other brain processes. Russian and British researchers report that carnosine improves learning and spacial orientation in experiments with rats. During these experiments, two groups of rats were exposed to severe ischaemia (i.e. they had the blood circulation to their brain blocked). One group had treatment with carnosine before the blood circulation was cut off and the other group did not receive any treatment. After the blood supply to the brain was cut off the researchers were surprised to find that a significant number of the carnosine-treated rats survived, and that the brain capability remained almost intact.

One explanation for this is that carnosine fine-tunes a chemical called glutamate or glutamic acid. Normally, glutamate binds onto certain brain cell receptors called NMDA (N-methyl-D-aspartate). This stimulates the release of nitric oxide which, in low amounts, arouses the brain and improves memory. By improving the supply of glutamate carnosine maintains the health of the brain, as shown in the above experiment with the rats. Too much glutamate, on the other hand, over-stimulates the NMDA receptor which causes overproduction of nitric oxide which, in turn, overexcites the brain. The whole process is made worse by free-floating zinc or copper metals. Carnosine, by binding to the zinc and copper metals modulates the NMDA receptor and calms things down.

Carnosine is a 'modulator', a word which is encountered frequently in anti-ageing research. A modulator is a sort of mediator which does two apparently simple things – it increases what is low, and it decreases what is high.

Carnosine and some of its relations (homocarnosine and acetyl-carnosine) activate other essential chemicals in the brain (for example sodium, potassium and adenosine tri-phosphate which is an energy chemical) and protect the brain cells against assault by free radicals. Overall, carnosine improves blood flow to the brain and reduces some lethal by-products of brain metabolism, bringing the brain metabolism into equilibrium.

Carnosine and Inflammation

One of the causes of ageing is chronic inflammation, as explained in the previous chapter. Chronic inflammation can be fuelled by excessive production of nitric oxide (NO), and I have already explained how excessive NO production may worsen brain function. Because carnosine reduces or blocks any excessive activity of NO, it may offer protection not only against oxidation and glycosylation, but also against the other age-related mechanism, that of chronic inflammation.

AGEs stimulate excessive production of NO and other toxic compounds, adding more poisonous ingredients to the already deadly soup of free radicals. By reducing AGEs, carnosine also lowers the production of these toxins. It will be obvious by now that all age-related processes are connected and depend on each other. When a protective agent such as carnosine acts in one area of ageing, this has repercussions further down the line, in other age-related processes.

Multiple Benefits

What do cancer, septic shock, asthma and migraines have in common? They are all associated with an increase in a special enzyme called guanylate cyclase. This enzyme is usually activated by NO and rises to sky-high levels in conditions like malignant tumours, severe sepsis, asthma and migraine attacks. Carnosine was shown to block the activation of guanylate cyclase and therefore can be of use in these conditions. More research is needed in this area, but initial results are promising.

By now you may be asking how such a simple molecule as carnosine can have so many diverse actions. Can it really be an antioxidant, a free radical scavenger, an anti-glycosylator, a chelator, and a membrane stabilizer used in diverse illnesses such as ulcers, cataracts, brain problems and diabetes? The answer is simple. Carnosine has some good properties itself, but when it is broken down by carnosinase, the resulting b-alanine and histidine have some advantages in their own right, as explained above. Adding to, or subtracting a few suitable chemical groups from the carnosine molecule, can result in other active products (for example, anserine, N-acetyl-carnosine, or carnosine–zinc complexes) with extra benefits on top of those of ordinary carnosine. So it is not just one compound we are dealing with but many related compounds which all work together to create many diverse results.

Is there any evidence behind the claims made for carnosine? There is, and plenty of it. In the following chapter I will present some of this evidence which demonstrates that carnosine is one of the best-studied anti-ageing nutrients available.

The Research Supporting Carnosine

The number of experiments exploring the diverse actions of carnosine is growing by the day. A great number of these experiments concentrate on the anti-glycosylating merits of carnosine and continue to discover more about its exact benefits. For example, in a recent experiment using sugars – such as glucose, fructose and ribose – and also aldehydes, Alan Hipkiss and his team at the University of London have shown that carnosine can protect against the injury these caused on muscle tissue. You might say that there is nothing new here and that we learned that from the previous chapter.

The surprising thing is that they have also discovered that certain other amino acids such as lysine and arginine, can protect against this type of injury too, but that their by-products, created when the reaction is over, may, on occasions, cause cancer. However, the by-products formed between the reaction of carnosine and sugars do not cause cancer. This shows us that there is still an enormous amount which needs to be learnt, not only about carnosine but also about any other nutrients which are claimed to have anti-ageing properties.

Human Clinical Trials

After evaluating and digesting the enormous amount of promising scientific information about the effects of carnosine in animals, I decided to start using carnosine for its anti-ageing value on humans. During the summer of 1999 I was the first clinical physician to use carnosine specifically for anti-ageing purposes on healthy human volunteers.

Since then I have been using various strengths of carnosine on many of my patients. Initial assessment of a small number of patients who took 50 mg–100 mg of carnosine a day showed that they experienced a variety of benefits. Some of their actual comments were:

- "It improved my clarity of thought."
- "People mention how well I look, and my sleep pattern is now normal."
- "It has improved my well-being, and my joints are more agile."
- "There has been a visible improvement in muscle tone, and a reduction of nocturnal cramps."
- "I have a heightened libido."
- "My sense of smell has improved."

Although several other patients did not report any obvious immediate benefits, most of them were willing to continue taking carnosine for general anti-ageing protection. No one has reported any side effects, even those who have been taking carnosine daily for over two years. These initial comments were quite encouraging and this made me want to go further, so I decided to study the effects of carnosine on the human body in more detail.

As I have already mentioned, MDA (malondialdehyde) is a toxic by-product, produced when free radicals attack lipids (fat), such as those found on the cell membrane. MDA starts its ugly work as soon as it is created, working hard to cross-link as many proteins as it can, but it is eventually eliminated in the urine.

There are tests which measure the levels of MDA in the urine and give an indication of the degree of destruction already caused by free radicals. There are, of course, many other toxic by-products of free radical metabolism but MDA is one of the most well studied. Several experiments done on animals show that carnosine inactivates and reduces the levels of this dangerous MDA. It is worth mentioning that the higher the amount of carnosine present, the lower the activity of the MDA, which is another way of saying that MDA and carnosine are extremely hostile to each other.

There is at least one home testing kit which measures urinary MDA. This is called the Vespro Free Radical Test (available from Vespro Ltd, see Useful Addresses). The patient collects some early morning urine, and mixes it with the special chemicals from the test kit. The results are then compared to a coloured chart. The colours correspond to four different values of MDA in the urine which, in turn, indicate four levels of free radical activity in the body, as follows:

- White corresponds to an extremely low MDA, showing an optimal level of free radicals working within the cells.
- Light pink corresponds to a low MDA level, and indicates a low free radical activity.
- Pink is for medium MDA levels corresponding to medium free radical activity.
- Dark pink means high MDA levels and a high free radical activity.

Because carnosine is able to neutralize MDA and protect the body tissues from it, the Free Radical Test is an ideal means of finding out whether taking carnosine supplements has any impact on the MDA concentration in your urine. Taking carnosine should help reduce the levels of MDA in the body, and this should be shown in the urine.

A Unique Trial

Based on this premise, I designed a clinical trial to research further. This is one of the first — perhaps the first — clinical trial to study the dosage and direct anti-ageing actions of carnosine on healthy humans. Because of this, I present all the details of the trial as they appeared in the official paperwork.

Does Oral Carnosine Supplementation Affect Urinary MDA?

AIM

To examine the effects of oral carnosine upon the concentration of urinary malondialdehyde (MDA), in everyday situations (i.e. outside laboratory conditions).

BACKGROUND

MDA is a product of lipid peroxidation which is also associated with age-related cross-linking of proteins and DNA. Carnosine is thought to:

1. Prevent lipid peroxidation and thus reduce MDA production
2. React with, and inactivate, existing MDA and thus also reduce MDA levels

Theoretically, introduction or withdrawal of carnosine supplementation should have a reducing or an increasing effect, respectively, on urinary MDA levels. This would possibly be a dose-dependent process.

MATERIALS AND METHODS

Oral L-carnosine (obtained from IAS/Pro-Found Products) was given to 20 healthy volunteers in a variety of dosages. This supplementation took place in addition to the participants' usual drug/supplement intake, which remained constant throughout the duration of the trial. Morning urine was collected and tested by the participants using a colorimetric test kit which measures urinary MDA concentrations (Vespro Free Radical Test)

PATIENTS

Male and female volunteers aged 40–75 were studied as follows:

A. Individuals who already were on carnosine were tested (day 1, baseline) and then asked to stop taking carnosine for one week. This was followed by a second urine test (day 8) and the carnosine supplementation was resumed. A final test was performed on day 15.

B. Individuals who were not on carnosine were tested at day 1, at day 8 (after using carnosine for a week) and at day 15 (after stopping carnosine for a week).

C. Individuals on increasing doses of carnosine were tested as follows: day 1 (baseline), day 8 (after taking carnosine 50 mg a day for a week), day 15 (after carnosine 100 mg a day for a week), day 21 (after carnosine 200 mg a day for a week)

D. The difference between a 50 mg and a 1000 mg daily dose was tested as follows: day 1 (baseline, no carnosine), day 8 (carnosine 50 mg), day 15 (carnosine 1000 mg)

DETAILS

The urine testing was performed in a 'single-blind' fashion, with only the examiner knowing the significance of the different colours. This was done in order to avoid patient-effected bias. The existing colours on the testing cards were numbered 1–4, and made available to the participants without any further details on their significance.

The results of the study were presented at the 2nd Monte Carlo Anti-Aging Conference in June 2001, and details were made available on a number of internet sites. The study has been peer-reviewed, and formal publication will follow.

RESULTS

In some volunteers a dose of as low as 50 mg a day was shown to have a measurable effect on the urinary MDA, improving it from 'high' to 'medium', or even to 'low'. Stopping carnosine for a week worsened MDA in two people. Others who did not experience any effects on 50 mg a day, were able to see a reduction in their MDA after increasing the carnosine to 100 mg–200 mg a day. Increasing the dose further, to 500 mg or even 1000 mg a day (in a limited number of volunteers) did not have any further effect on MDA, i.e. it did not improve the beneficial results already experienced while on 100–200 mg a day.

This shows that it is not necessary to take high doses of carnosine to overcome its destruction by carnosinases, and even 50 mg a day is effective in some people, particularly perhaps in those who have a genetic predisposition to a low activity of carnosinase. Overall, the ideal dose was found to be around 100 mg to 150 mg a day. It is preferable to use co-enzyme Q10 and vitamin E together with carnosine, as many volunteers who were taking these two supplements experienced a quicker improvement of their MDA levels.

Those volunteers who exercised heavily showed the worst initial results, having an increased MDA which indicates an increased activity of free radicals during exercise.

Some other volunteers who took carnosine did not show any changes in their MDA, and this could be due to having an increased carnosinase activity which destroyed carnosine before it could have any effects. However, these are very early stages and no firm conclusions can be made regarding this. More research is planned using higher doses of carnosine.

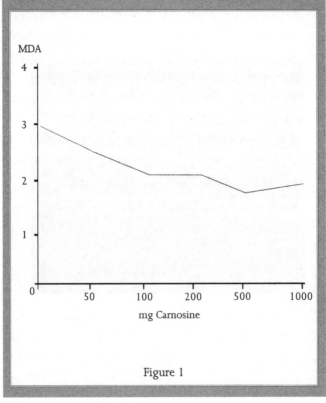

Figure 1

The Use of Carnosine for Specific Illnesses

Over the years carnosine has been used to treat different illnesses, from arthritis and high blood pressure to ulcers and inflammation. The following are examples of clinical conditions treated with carnosine.

ARTHRITIS and BONE HEALTH

It was some pioneering Polish doctors who first used carnosine specifically for improving joint health, nearly 60 years ago. At that time, doctors recorded encouraging results, including improvement of the symptoms of rheumatoid arthritis. The treatment was given by injection (0.5 mg–1 mg every other day). These early studies also showed a clear improvement of components of the blood which are usually connected with inflammation (for example ESR, or the erythrocyte sedimentation rate, and eosinophilic cells). The carnosine treatment was particularly effective when combined with physiotherapy. These experiments were later confirmed by other researchers, who used high doses of carnosine.

More recently, Japanese researchers experimenting with carnosine–zinc combinations on post-menopausal women who have rheumatoid arthritis, found that this treatment reduces the severity of the symptoms. Their research showed that the carnosine–zinc combination reduces pain and strengthens the bone structure in the wrists, probably by stimulating the bone-forming cells, called osteoblasts, to produce new and healthy bone tissue. These are promising results, but we are still some way from seeing carnosine taking its place among the conventional, run-of-the-mill anti-arthritic drugs.

HIGH BLOOD PRESSURE

During experiments with cats and dogs, carnosine given by injection over 15 days was able to lower blood pressure quite significantly. This was also shown to be the case by Russian scientists in a few unconfirmed reports in humans. The reason why carnosine has not become a popular treatment for high blood pressure is that there are other more potent drugs available. It is interesting to note that the drug ALT711 (which will be discussed later on) is also thought to be able to reduce high blood pressure. Carnosine and ALT711 have similar actions, in that they both reduce the damage caused by glycosylation on the wall of the arteries, which then thickens the arteries and eventually results in high blood pressure.

In addition, carnosine has the extra bonus of being able to modulate NO (nitric oxide). Nitric oxide, in the right amounts relaxes the arteries, thus reducing high blood pressure. Incidentally, NO also increases blood circulation to the penis. Indeed Viagra works by balancing NO, with the well known uplifting results. Carnosine may also have a positive effect on erections, through its NO balancing acts, but this has not yet been studied in detail.

BLOOD CLOTTING

Platelets are small constituents of the blood which play an active part in blood clotting. If, for some reason, they clump together too much, they cause an excessive clotting of the blood, which may result in a blockage of the artery, manifesting as a stroke, for example. If the platelets are a bit sluggish at clumping together, then the result is defective clotting of the blood with consequent haemorrhage. Carnosine has been shown to be able to modulate and regulate the action of platelets and in this way it balances blood clotting. In patients with abnormally quick clotting of the blood, carnosine decreases the clumping of the platelets, thus preventing stroke. In those patients who have an inability to control excessive bleeding, it does the opposite, stimulating the platelets to clump together and thus reduce bleeding.

ULCERS

Carnosine stimulates the formation of new skin (epithelium) over gastric ulcers, and stimulates other organs such as the liver and pancreas which, in turn, influence the workings of the stomach. Seeing an excellent opportunity, some entrepreneurial Japanese researchers have developed a carnosine–zinc combination, along the lines discussed in the previous chapter, with the brand name Polaprezinc. This is officially approved in Japan for the treatment of stomach and duodenal ulcers. When taken in tablet form, Polaprezinc remains inside the stomach for a relatively long time to cover the ulcer, after which the carnosine and the zinc dissolve and start healing the ulcer. Simple and effective.

These researchers have shown that the carnosine–zinc compound reduces the damage caused by the bacterium helicobacter pylori on the stomach. Helicobacter pylori is a bacterium present in your stomach which, if allowed to multiply beyond a certain critical point, causes ulcers. The current conventional treatment for helicobacter pylori is with a combination of antibiotics and anti-acid drugs, but if carnosine is proven to reduce this bacterium in further trials it may well become a standard, worldwide treatment for ulcers. Polaprezinc is definitely a company to watch.

Polaprezinc has also been reported to be a strong antioxidant protecting the lining of the stomach. During an experiment performed at the Keio University in Tokyo, Japan, it was shown that acid in the stomach causes extensive disruption of the DNA content of the stomach cells, but that Polaprezinc was able to reduce this.

WOUNDS AND SKIN HEALTH

It is a fact that applying carnosine directly on wounds speeds up the healing of the skin, without producing an exaggerated amount of collagen, which means that there is no excessive scarring. Brazilian and Japanese researchers have shown that carnosine speeds up production of granulation tissue, which is the healing material that fills a wound, just like cement fills in cracks in a wall. In another experiment, when carnosine was added to a nutritious formula given to people who had extensive wounds, it improved the rate of wound healing and it stimulated the natural mechanisms of repair.

Due to its anti-glycosylating properties, carnosine protects the collagen and elastin molecules in the skin. These are necessary molecules which give the skin its smooth, firm appearance. Other constituents of the skin – for example the fibroblasts and the material between the cells and the collagen which is called the 'extracellular matrix' – are also protected by carnosine. This is why Australians introduced carnosine cream for anti-ageing skin care. They market their products under the trade name Beta Alistine. Clinical trials with this particular form of carnosine are still necessary to prove its effectiveness.

AN UNUSUAL ANTI-INFLAMMATORY

I am always surprised by the different ways a remedy can be used. So I was intrigued to find out that carnosine can be used in toothpaste. If used in this form, it was found to be an effective treatment for inflammation of the gums. It suppresses an excessive immune reaction and stimulates a sluggish one, bringing the system back to normal equilibrium. It activates and protects immune cells (called B cells and T cells) which are necessary in controlling inflammation.

Another unusual way of using carnosine is by nasal spray. Carnosine has a particular affinity for the olfactory nerve and can easily go from the nose, via the smell nerve, straight into the brain, stimulating it and protecting it. Before you rush out to buy these carnosine sprays, I have to tell you that they are still in the experimental form and not yet generally available for the public.

CANCER

High doses of carnosine (1000 mg–3000 mg in tablet form, daily) have been used by Russian doctors to treat inoperable tumours, and to protect against the effects of radiotherapy or chemotherapy. In experiments using such high doses in humans, carnosine showed both short-term and long-term improvements, such as protecting against an excessive lowering of valuable white blood cells, the concentration of which usually plummets during chemotherapy or radiotherapy. It also stabilized the cell membrane after it was damaged by radiation. Cancer cells increase sugar production because they need the chemical energy from the sugar in order to survive. Carnosine blocks this by reducing sugar availability, and therefore it has the potential to starve cancer cells to death, by blocking their energy supply.

INCREASED LIFESPAN

The results of an experiment showed that mice fed on high doses of carnosine live, on average, 20% longer than mice fed on ordinary food. In other similar experiments it was shown that the average lifespan increases and that an increased number of animals live to reach old age. However, the maximum lifespan is not affected. The maximum lifespan is the maximum number of years (or months, from the mice point of view) that can ever be achieved, whereas the average lifespan is the average length of time people (or mice) actually live.

In a combined Russian-British experiment, the following changes were observed in mice fed on carnosine:

- improved glossiness of their fur
- a better ability to heal skin ulcers
- an improved posture.

After another series of experiments, Australian researchers led by Dr Robin Holliday from Sydney, reported that carnosine extends the lifespan of human cells in the laboratory. Human fibroblasts are special cells typically present in the skin and they play a part in creating new collagen molecules. When physiological (i.e. normal, not excessive) amounts of carnosine are added to a mixture of these cells in the laboratory they live for about 20% longer, which corresponds nicely with the mice experiments discussed above.

These cells also become able to divide more times than usual. Normally fibroblasts can divide around 50 times after which they become unable to divide any longer and so they die. This is called the Hayflick limit, after Leonard Hayflick who first described the phenomenon back in the early 60s. His theories suggest that it is impossible to overcome this limit and therefore we are restricted as to the amount of time we can live. During the Australian experiments, however, it was shown that this is not true, because fibroblasts treated with carnosine could divide an average of 60 times, and sometimes up to 70 times, well above the Hayflick limit.

During further experiments, scientists where able to test fibroblast cells taken from human foreskin and from human lung tissue. The addition of carnosine to the fibroblasts was found to restore these cells to a more youthful appearance. Let me explain this in some more detail. With age, fibroblasts in a laboratory environment lose their normal, youthful characteristics. For example:

- they fail to line up in parallel lines
- they become irregular in size and shape
- there is a build up of debris and empty spaces, called 'vacuoles', inside the fibroblast cell.

Carnosine reverses all of these age-related changes, making the fibroblasts behave like younger cells, making them look regular in shape and size, and arrange themselves in straight lines.

Other experiments confirmed that, apart from having their Hayflick limit extended, carnosine-treated fibroblasts were able to live to over 400 days, instead of the normal 310. A different variant of these experiments showed that cells were able to keep on dividing to live 413 days, whereas similar cells not treated with carnosine died after an average of 132 days. All of these results were seen in cells treated with normal amounts of carnosine as low as those normally found in living muscle tissue (i.e. not excessively high). These experiments also show that normal amounts of carnosine are slightly better than marginally higher amounts. In technical terms, 20mM concentrations of carnosine extend cell divisions to a total of 70 cell doublings, whereas concentrations of 30mM can only extend the divisions up to 64 doublings.

Ageing goes hand in hand with telomere shortening. Telomeres are parts of the DNA molecule – at the end of the molecule – which are usually long, protecting the DNA against defects during replication (i.e. during the division of DNA to create two daughter molecules of DNA). With age, the telomeres become progressively shorter and thus less effective, until the DNA cannot function any longer, eventually destroying the cell. Free radical and other toxins accelerate the shrinkage of telomeres. Once damaged, the telomeres are almost impossible to repair. It would make biological sense if antioxidants could effectively protect the telomeres from free radical damage before this happens. It turns out that only carnosine is capable of this protective action, out of all the other antioxidants tested so far.

It is worth reminding you that there is a difference between experiments in animals and those in humans, but the initial results on carnosine are very encouraging indeed. Carnosine is one of the most promising nutrients which may help people to achieve their maximum lifespan potential, and increase the percentage of people who become centenarians. Carnosine was discovered just over 100 years ago and by using it this may be an age that most people should aim to reach.

Clear Vision

I am now going to discuss what carnosine can do to your eyes. One of its most exciting properties is its ability to treat cataract.

Cataract is a very common cause of blindness worldwide, affecting over 17 million people. This is over half of the world's blind population. 'Cataract' is Greek for 'waterfall', and this describes the difficulty for patients who see things as if they are behind a waterfall. The conventional treatment of cataract is by special glasses initially, and then by surgical removal of the affected lens followed by a transplant with a new, artificial one. Taking antioxidants has been advised by some doctors to try and prevent further impairment to the eye, but this does nothing to reverse an already existing cataract.

There are different types of cataract which affect different parts of the lens. The lens of the eye is formed by fibres — strings of proteins and other chemicals — which are transparent, allowing the light to reach the inside of the eye and create a visual image. Free radicals which are active within the lens destroy the fibres, initiating changes that lead to cataract. For example, free radicals speed up the destruction of biological membranes and of certain valuable proteins inside the lens, called crystallins. Damaged crystallins do not allow much light to pass through and this results in poor vision.

Normally the crystallins and other components of the lens are protected against free radicals by a strong presence of antioxidants such as glutathione, which is a very effective free radical quencher, as well as vitamins A and E and carnosine. However, increasing age reduces these antioxidants in the lens leaving it without much protection. When this happens, damaged crystallins inside the lens accumulate and cause a 'clouding over' of the lens which leads to the state of affairs known as 'cataract'.

This is where carnosine comes in. Normally carnosine is present inside the lens in large amounts, which means that it has a natural role to play in protecting against the progression of lens damage. When cataract develops carnosine becomes severely deficient in the lens. Some people believe that this means that, when carnosine is low in the lens, cataract becomes inescapable.

One way carnosine works is by removing the peroxide compounds which are the leftover toxic products following damage to the cell membrane. Carnosine, and its relative N-alpha-acetyl-carnosine, not only have antioxidant benefits of their own but also boost the action of other antioxidants in the lens such as that of glutathione.

Experiments with rabbits show that adding a carnosine preparation to the lens increases the carnosine content inside the lens, i.e. carnosine is able to reach the lens if given externally in eye drops. Carnosine can delve deep into the lens and even reach parts of the lens which other antioxidants are unable to reach as, for example, in posterior subcapsular cataract. This has been debated by some scientists who think that the variant N-alpha-acetyl-carnosine is much more able to penetrate the lens than ordinary carnosine.

Apart from free radical protection of the lens, carnosine is also active against glycosylation. Glycosylation inside the lens causes abnormal bonds between proteins and sugar molecules, creating thick and twisted proteins which are not transparent. With time, more and more proteins accumulate, causing the characteristic clouding over of the lens and consequent loss of vision. Because carnosine is a strong anti-glycosylator, it has been used as a serious anti-cataract agent.

One of the things that speed up the formation of cataract is radiation, typically ultraviolet (UV) radiation from the sun, but perhaps also radiation from mobile telephones, computer screens and even television screens. In experiments with lens extracts in the laboratory, when the lens was exposed to bright light for long periods, the production of abnormal proteins was speeded up which caused the early changes typical of cataract. In animals exposure to strong sunlight was found to have similar results. UV radiation causes a lethal cocktail of free radicals with names like superoxide anion, hydroxyl radical, singlet oxygen and lipid peroxide. All of these destroy the constituents of the lens, as explained above, resulting in cataract.

With regards to injury caused by artificial radiation from mobile telephones, this is thought to play a role in accelerating cataract but there is no agreement between scientists as to whether this is a real or an insignificant risk. It may be best to be on the safe side, however, and to consider the use of a phone shield and antioxidants, including carnosine, for any eventuality.

It has to be said that cataract is a very complicated process involving many other mechanisms which have not been studied in detail. Free radicals, glycosylation and UV radiation, as well as several immune reactions play an important role in the formation of cataract, but there are other processes which need to be considered and clarified.

However, because carnosine is active against so many different processes, it is being used to deal with the problems caused by cataract. Several experiments with dogs suffering from age-related cataract have shown the positive effects of carnosine in improving the condition. Note that I said 'improving' and not merely 'preventing'. Improving means that the damage was already done and carnosine has repaired it, has reversed it. In these experiments with dogs, when treatment with carnosine eye drops was continued for four months, the cataract improvement was sustained, i.e. there was no worsening of the condition.

In an experiment by Russian researchers in 1997 involving 109 human patients, carnosine eye drops at a concentration of 5%, were also found to be effective in healing eye infections such as keratitis, and other eye conditions such as corneal erosions, corneal dystrophy and keratopathy, and corneal ulcers due to herpes, and bacterial infections. This is probably due to carnosine's ability to stimulate the repair processes inside the eye.

In another experiment, a carnosine derivative was found to be able to reduce intraocular pressure. High intraocular pressure (i.e. pressure of fluid inside the eye) is related to glaucoma, so in theory carnosine could help patients with this condition, although further research is needed here. The Pharmacological Committee of the Russian Ministry of Health has approved carnosine eye drops for the treatment of medical eye conditions.

Carnosine as it stands may be unable to stay in the eye tissues for long because it is inactivated by carnosinase. For this reason, a stronger and more difficult to destroy form of carnosine has been developed called N-alpha-acetyl-carnosine (NACA). This is basically carnosine fortified with a special chemical group called acetyl. NACA is not as strong as carnosine when it comes to antioxidant action, but it lasts longer in the tissues.

During recent years, researchers have been able to show that NACA eye drops reverse the symptoms of cataract in humans. This form of carnosine can remain in the lens for quite some time and therefore can exert its benefits over a long period. In a classic experiment, Russian and American scientists studied 49 people with an average age of 65 years, who had been diagnosed with age-related cataract. Half of the patients were treated with NACA eye drops, and the other half were not treated, but only used for comparison purposes.

After six months of treatment, over 40% of the carnosine-treated patients experienced an improvement in the transmission of light through the lens, and almost 90% of these patients were found to experience up to 100% improvement of vision and sensitivity to glare. Sensitivity to glare increases with normal ageing, due to light being scattered by the non-transparent lens.

After 24 months of treatment these benefits were still continuing. In other words, as long as the treatment continued, the patients were protected against age-related cataract. The control patients (those who were not treated with carnosine), experienced a normal worsening of vision as would have been expected in anybody of that age. No significant side effects were reported in this study. The researchers concluded that the acetylated form of carnosine (N-alpha-acetyl-carnosine) is a suitable non-surgical treatment for age-related cataract.

The results of this experiment are far-reaching, suggesting that cataract could not only be prevented but also cured with simple eye drops. The same researchers have found similar results in earlier experiments with rabbits, and their results on humans have also been replicated by Chinese researchers.

During a preliminary communication I had with Dr Aimin Wang of the Harbin Medical University in China, he explained his clinical trials which showed that carnosine cures age-related cataract. In two experiments in 1997 and 1999, he and his co-workers studied 96 patients, whose average age was 60 years, with age-related cataract. They used 1–2 drops of carnosine in each eye, 3–4 times a day for up to 6 months. They found that the carnosine-treated patients experienced an improvement of their condition at an amazing cure rate of 80–100%, with no side effects. This ties in with what the Russians have found in the experiments mentioned above. In another trial, Dr Wang studied 1000 patients with cataract and found similar benefits. His team also used carnosine drops in other eye conditions and found it to be effective in improving general eyesight, giving clear vision and brightening the eyes.

Following these pioneering experiments, carnosine eye drops are now used commercially, as a treatment of cataract. Results of ongoing studies are awaited to confirm the benefits beyond doubt. There is a debate as to which form of carnosine is the best to use in cataract. Some researchers say that the NACA form is best because ordinary carnosine may be transformed into histamine in the eye and cause toxicity. I did explain the benefits and drawbacks of histamine in the previous chapter, but the problem is that we still do not know whether histamine can cause toxicity in the eye tissues specifically. In other words, we do not know whether the actions of carnosine as described for other parts of the body, also hold true for the eye. Until the issue is clarified, it may be best to choose eye drops in the NACA form in preference to ordinary carnosine.

Carnosinemia

I know some people who are reluctant to use carnosine, as they are concerned about a condition called 'carnosinemia', which means too much carnosine in the blood. They fear that carnosine can be toxic and cause dramatic side effects such as:

- mental retardation
- muscle paralysis
- fits and blindness.

These, however, are the consequences of a serious and rare genetic condition, related to a defective chromosome 18. In this disease, the enzyme carnosinase is absent from the body, leaving carnosine to accumulate in extremely high amounts and cause serious side effects. The excess carnosine is then eliminated in the urine. This condition is not found in people who take carnosine only for anti-ageing purposes. The very few people who are unfortunate enough to have carnosinemia, will have known about it from childhood.

There are people, however, who may have a generally weak activity of carnosinase, leaving mildly increased amounts of carnosine in the body. These people are the most liable to suffer from very mild side effects after taking large amounts of supplemental carnosine. On the other hand, some people may have a stronger activity of carnosinase, which destroys carnosine at a relatively brisker pace, and so they may need to take slightly higher amounts of carnosine, in order to compensate. There is no commercial way of testing whether one has high or low carnosinase activity, so people who take carnosine supplements do so on a 'trial and error' basis. This is one of the reasons why I strongly recommend using carnosine only under medical supervision.

Purity

Several early trials evaluating the effects of carnosine were flawed because impure carnosine preparations were used. Even recently there have been concerns about the purity of commercially available carnosine which was contaminated with the chemical hydrazine which can be toxic if used in large amounts. It commonly contaminates synthetic carnosine, and makes some of the benefits of carnosine more difficult to study.

Some scientists believe that at least some of the benefits ascribed to carnosine are not due to carnosine at all but due to the presence of hydrazine contaminating the mixture. This is somewhat far-fetched, but it highlights the importance of using carnosine from reputable sources, to avoid the risk of side effects due to hydrazine or other contaminants.

A Carnosine-Rich Diet

For those people who want to enjoy some of the benefits of carnosine without taking supplements in tablet form, it is possible to follow a diet rich in natural carnosine. Carnosine is found in red meat and chicken, particularly chicken breast. It is also present in eyes and nervous tissue, so those who, like the Japanese, eat fish eyes may be getting a good share of carnosine.

Reasonable amounts of carnosine are also found in sprinting game such as rabbits and hares, and in other poultry such as pheasant. This corresponds with current nutritional advice which recommends choosing game meat as being healthier than hormonally-treated pork or beef. Carnosine is not found in any fruit or vegetables. This is not surprising as the prefix 'carn-' in carnosine, comes from the Latin meaning 'meat' or 'flesh'.

Who Should be Taking Carnosine?

Carnosine supplements are ideal for three things:

1. General anti-ageing protection. Out of the five main causes of ageing, carnosine deals with oxidation, glycosylation and chronic inflammation, as well as being a potential hormonal receptor regulator.
2. Prevention of diseases such as cataract, cancer, muscle weakness, heart disease, diabetes and dementia
3. Specific treatment of existing conditions such as cataract, ulcers, and diabetic complications under medical supervision, in higher doses than usual.

Dosage

There has been a lot of speculation regarding the exact dose of carnosine. The Life Extension Foundation in the United States recommends an average of 1000 mg a day (500 mg–1500 mg) of carnosine in order to overcome the destruction by carnosinase and leave some carnosine free to work on the body. They extrapolated this dosage from the dosage of carnosine used in radiation protection experiments with mice.

During those experiments a maximum oral daily dose of carnosine of 500 mg per kg of body weight was used, which is the equivalent of 35000 mg a day for an average human. In some Russian experiments with cancer patients undergoing radiotherapy a dose of 3000 mg was used. This, however, was aimed at treating radiotherapy damage, and so the high dose has no bearing on an average healthy person, who just wants to get some protection against ageing processes. Questions remain as to whether such high doses are really necessary.

In rats, positive results were seen with doses of as little as 2 mg per kg of body weight, the equivalent of around 150 mg for an average human. No toxic side effects were seen even when the dose was increased to 500 mg per kg of body weight. Remember that these doses are for rats and not humans.

As I have already explained, during preliminary clinical trials I performed with carnosine, a dose of 100 mg–150 mg a day was sufficient to affect MDA levels and the argument for the need to flood the carnosinase system with carnosine does not appear valid. As little as 50 mg of carnosine a day may effect measurable changes in the body.

However, there are clinical trials in progress using high doses of carnosine, trying to establish whether the 1000 mg dose is better than the 100 mg one. At the moment, as things stand, I think that the arguments support the lower dose (50 mg–150 mg a day) but this may well change in favour of the higher dose (1000 mg) when results of ongoing experiments are released.

Carnosine is cheap and is becoming readily available. It is best to take carnosine together with vitamin E and co-enzyme Q10 for ideal protection. Almost all other nutrients can also be taken with carnosine and there are no adverse effects reported with carnosine interacting with other drugs or nutrients. Carnosine is now available mixed with vodka (80 mg per 200 ml). The vodka enhances carnosine absorption from the bowel. In turn, carnosine protects the liver against the effect of the vodka. Carnosine is also being made available in a toothpaste form for healthy, infection-free gums. Finally, it is soon to be manufactured in the spray form for inhalation through the nose. This way of taking carnosine ensures that it reaches the brain directly through the olfactory nerve, without being destroyed by carnosinase.

Side Effects

No side effects have been recorded, apart from rare muscular problems, such as mild trembling and occasional allergic reactions (blocked sinuses), when using a very high dose of carnosine (1000 mg a day). One of the main problems frequently encountered by carnosine users is that it may not have obvious immediate benefits for everyone. It is necessary for carnosine to be used for years to gain sustained anti-ageing protection, and the results may not be evident in the short term.

Other Anti-glycosylators

The normal ageing process causes loss of collagen and elastic fibres, by glycosylation, not only of the skin but also of the heart and arteries. Chemicals that prevent or reverse glycosylation are therefore thought to be important in reversing ageing changes. Carnosine is one of these chemicals, but there are several others.

ALT711

A company called Alteon Corporation in the United States is researching several anti-glycosylators. Their most important product is ALT711 (a thiazolium salt with the chemical name: 4,5 dimethyl-3-phenacyl-thiazolium chloride). This has been used in experiments to reverse problems such as thickening and loss of elasticity of the heart, and of the arteries, and it reduces blood pressure and improves circulation.

Experiments with dogs show that ALT711 reverses age-related stiffness of the arteries by 40%, and improves cardiac function. Carnosine and similar products prevent cross-linking, but ALT711 actually breaks the bonds between already cross-linked proteins, i.e. after cross-linking has already taken place. The action of ALT711 is definite proof that damage from at least one basic biological ageing process can indeed be reversed. There are other 'cross-link breakers' such as PTB (phenacyl-thiazolium bromide), similar to ALT711, but these are not as well studied as it is.

There is no clear evidence at present to show whether carnosine can indeed break existing bonds, just like

ALT711. Some researchers believe that this is quite possible, perhaps due to the ability of carnosine to increase glutathione which interferes with a certain type of chemical bond (called S–S bonds) on the cross-linked proteins. Carnosine is able to remove already cross-linked proteins, however, and so it leaves the cells unobstructed to form new and healthy proteins.

To give you an analogy, think of a cross-linked protein as a house hit by a small bomb. ALT711 can repair the damage and make the house appear brand new again. Carnosine prevents the bomb from falling in the first place, plus it bulldozes any already damaged houses to the ground and clears the rubbish, leaving the place free for a new house to be built. Ideally, carnosine and ALT711 could, in theory, be taken together to complement each other's actions. In fact carnosine *should* be taken together with ALT711 because, when ALT711 breaks the bonds between the two cross-linked proteins, these are liable to reattach to each other again, and so carnosine is necessary to prevent them from cross-linking again. Otherwise we would be back where we started. At the time of writing, ALT711 is not yet available to the general public.

AMINOGUANIDINE

Also marketed as Pimagedine, this is a typical anti-glycosylator. It prevents cross-linking but does not affect bonds already formed between proteins. Its actions are somewhat similar to those of carnosine. For example, it can inactivate carbonyl groups on proteins and so reduce the risk of cross-linking. It also reduces toxic aldehydes and it is therefore effective during the early stages of glycosylation. One of its actions is to protect the kidneys against glycosylation, and human experiments show that aminoguanidine reduces the amount of useful protein lost in the urine.

Other potential benefits are seen in diabetes, where it helps stabilize the blood glucose, as well as reducing LDL cholesterol. It increases the collagen scaffolding within the arterial walls of older people by 30%, thus strengthening the arteries. Side effects are limited to mild nausea and headache. The hydrochloride form of aminoguanidine, although more expensive, is preferable to the bicarbonate form which is difficult for the body to assimilate. The suggested dose is 150 mg–450 mg a day, divided into two or three doses.

TENISLETAM

This drug was first used as an anti-anginal drug and then as a brain booster. It inhibits cross-linking and it has been found to have some positive results in Alzheimer's disease, by reducing the amount of dangerous beta amyloid in the brain. It works by blocking the sites where proteins can be cross-linked, and so it has an action similar to that of carnosine and aminoguanidine. The current consensus is that it does not break existing bonds like ALT711 does.

PYRIDOXAMINE

Pyridorin is the brand name of pyridoxamine, a derivative of vitamin B6 (pyridoxine). It is a potent inhibitor of cross-linking and an AGE preventor. It also has some anti-oxidation properties. It prevents free radical damage to sugar molecules, and so it prevents sugar molecules from being activated to initiate glycosylation.

Pyridoxamine inactivates carbonyl groups, just like the other compounds mentioned above, and it is particularly effective in the later stages of glycosylation. It could turn out to have clinical benefits in diabetes and atherosclerosis and is currently being evaluated by the manufacturers of Pyridorin, who are planning to license it as a drug, needing a doctor's prescription and not as a nutrient. This is because the manufacturers want to make sure that it has no toxic side effects, particularly if used in high doses.

REFERENCES

1. Kyriazis M. 'Carnosine, the new anti-aging supplement'. *Anti-aging Bulletin* 2000, 4(6):3–7.

2. Kyriazis M. 'The difference between NAC and L-carnosine'. *Anti-aging Bulletin* 2001, 4(11):18–24.

3. Quinn P., Boldyrev A, 'Carnosine: its properties, functions and potential therapeutic applications'. *Molecular Aspects of Medicine* 1992, 13:379–444.

4. Ukeda H. et al. 'Effect of carnosine and related compounds on the inactivation of human Cu, Zn–SOD'. *Bioscience, Biotechnology and Biochemistry* 2002, 66(1):36–43.

5. Hipkiss A. et al. 'Reaction of carnosine with aged proteins'. *Ann NY Ac Sci* 2002, 959:285–294.

6. Hyland P., Duggan O., Hipkiss A. 'The effects of carnosine on oxidative DNA damage'. *Mech Ageing Dev* 2000, 121(1–3):203–215.

7. Gariballa S., Sinclair A. 'Carnosine: physiological properties and therapeutic potential'. *Age Ageing* 2000, 29:207–210.

8. Hipkiss A. 'Carnosine, a protective, anti-ageing peptide?' *International Journal of Biochemistry and Cell Biology* 1998, 30:863–868.

9. Babizhayev M. et al. 'Imidazole-containing peptido-mimetic NACA'. *Journal of Anti Aging Medicine* 2000, 3(1):43–61.

10. Wang A. et al. 'Use of carnosine as a natural anti-senescence drug for human beings'. *Biochemistry* 2000, 65(7):869–871.

11. Yamano T. et al. 'Effect of carnosine on hyperglycaemia'. *Neurosci Lett* 2001, 313(1–2):78–82.

DHEA

If carnosine is nature's answer to glycosylation, what about the other processes of ageing? How can we fight oxidation, methylation, inflammation and hormonal imbalance?

Let us take one thing at a time. In the following two chapters, I will consider two main hormones (DHEA and growth hormone) which are used to improve age-related hormonal imbalance. In chapter 6, it is the turn of the anti-oxidant co-enzyme Q10 to go under the microscope, while in chapter 7 I will introduce you to a few methylation-boosting nutrients. All of the above substances also have certain beneficial effects on inflammation, and I will highlight these where appropriate.

So, what is DHEA? DHEA stands for De-Hydro-Epi-Androsterone, although it could easily stand for 'don't hasten early ageing'. It is a hormone produced by the adrenal glands (small organs snuggled up near the kidneys) and it is created by a chemical reaction involving the dreaded cholesterol molecule. Cholesterol is not always up to mischief, but can sometimes behave itself and be of some use to you. DHEA is an essential starting point for the production of other hormones such as oestrogen and progesterone (the 'female' hormones) and testosterone (the 'male' hormone). It circulates in the blood under the form of DHEA-Sulphate, which is inactive, and needs to be reactivated by the cells into DHEA proper before it can start its good deeds.

Like several other hormones, its production goes down through the floor with the passage of time. This fall starts from one's early twenties and continues throughout middle age. In some instances its levels fall to a meagre 30% of the youthful levels, and this is just at the age of 40–50. As I mentioned at the beginning of this book, a fall of a particular hormone with age may not necessarily be a bad thing, it may just be the way Mother Nature prepares you to deal with the rigours of ageing. However, it is becoming increasingly clear that this may not the case with DHEA. Falling DHEA levels are associated with a number of illnesses which are connected to ageing.

Scientific Trials

Although anti-ageing treatment with DHEA has been around for many years, it gained some scientific acceptance only in 1995, when the New York Academy of Sciences published a prestigious book summarizing all the positive points of DHEA. There are over 2000 scientific studies (most on animals, some on humans) which show that it has a positive role to play in ageing.

For example, in a study performed at the University of California it was shown that taking 50 mg of DHEA every day for six months, pushes the DHEA levels in the blood right up to those of youth. Up to 84% of women and 67% of men who took part in this particular study reported that the treatment made them feel better, both physically and mentally. When the dose was increased to 100 mg a day, in men only, their muscle strength and muscle tissue improved considerably. At that dose, their insulin growth factor 1 (IGF1) levels were also improved. As I will discuss in chapter 5, this IGF1 is an important hormone intermediary which is responsible for improving muscle tissue, reducing fat and boosting the immune system – a really useful hormone.

A particular form of DHEA called '7-keto DHEA' is believed to be more stable and about 2–3 times stronger than the real thing. The 7-keto variety does not easily convert to oestrogen or testosterone and so it may be useful to those who want to avoid the side effects related to these two hormones. 7-keto also has a more powerful beneficial effect on the immune system. Animal experiments with the 7-keto variety did not show any significant side effects even at doses equivalent to a whopping 140 times the normal dose for humans.

During a highly publicized recent experiment, French Professor E. Baulieu and co-workers studied 280 healthy older people aged 60–79. Half of these people were given 50 mg of DHEA every day for a year, whereas the other half only took a placebo, or dummy pill. This clinical trial was therefore handled correctly in that it was a double blind, placebo-controlled study, which is the highest standard of respectable scientific research methods. These are the results in those patients who were treated with DHEA:

- there were no obvious harmful side effects
- the concentration of DHEA in the blood returned to younger (higher) levels
- a small increase in testosterone/oestrogen was noted, equivalent to the benefits of mild HRT
- the production of new bone tissue increased in women over 70 years old
- there was a significant increase in libido in these women
- all the participants, but particularly the women, experienced an improved skin health, with skin thickness and hydration increasing, and age-pigments reducing.

This is a serious supporting scientific study, which should allay any fears about side effects or about DHEA not being active or useful. As mentioned previously however, this treatment does not turn the ageing clock back, but merely improves the external and internal appearance of the user.

In an even more rigorous study, a double-blind, cross-over, placebo-controlled clinical trial (see the glossary for an explanation of these terms) people aged 40–70 were given either 50mg of DHEA a day or a placebo. Over 80% of those who took the DHEA reported an improved quality of sleep, better mental and physical well-being and an improved ability to handle stress, compared to only 10%

improvement reported by those who took dummy treatment.

Facts about DHEA

- It increases antioxidant activity in rabbits and, possibly, in humans.
- It activates osteoblasts, the bone-forming cells.
- It protects against LDL (the 'bad' fat), particularly in older people and thus reduces the risk of heart disease.

Some Other Benefits of DHEA

IMMUNE BOOSTER

Several experiments show that DHEA is able to keep chronic inflammation under control. Chronic inflammation is thought to be involved in causing illnesses such as Alzheimer's disease, arthritis, brain failure, heart disease, and kidney disease. DHEA is found to help reduce the effects of chronic inflammation in a variety of ways. For example, it reduces interleukin 6 (IL6) which is a chemical frequently found in immune diseases such as rheumatoid arthritis. IL6 levels increase with age and measuring IL6 is, in fact, a guide as to how quickly the body ages. In double-blind cross-over studies, 50 mg of DHEA was found to reduce IL6 and improve the actions of natural killer cells which are essential in eliminating foreign viruses or bacteria. DHEA also encourages the production of interferon which is a substance needed for fighting several inflammatory disorders. Interferon is most notably used in some cases of multiple sclerosis.

On the other hand, studies have also highlighted the negative side of DHEA. For example it does nothing to boost the immune system against influenza in older people. Others believe that high doses of DHEA may actually worsen the risk of some cancers such as those of the prostate or the breast.

HORMONES

DHEA increases IGF1 (an intermediary of growth hormone) by about 10%. You can see how one hormone like DHEA can influence another apparently unrelated one – growth hormone. In this particular case, the end result may well turn out to be a lowering of the risk of osteoporosis, because IGF1 stimulates the activity of osteoblasts – cells which form new bone. DHEA is also used in slowing the progress of certain cancers (except those of the prostate and the breast), but that treatment is, of course, undertaken under strict medical supervision.

BRAIN HEALTH

Some experts believe that damage to the nerves happens at a faster rate when DHEA levels are low. In experiments, adding DHEA to nerve cells in the laboratory can make them stronger and better able to withstand chemical and toxic assault. In mice DHEA treatment improves memory and helps them remember their way around a maze. DHEA levels are about

50% lower in the brain of Alzheimer's dementia patients compared to healthy people of a similar age, and so it is now being used in experiments with humans to determine whether it has any definite beneficial effects on dementia. DHEA protects brain cells against excitotoxicity and against the formation of beta amyloid, a substance which I have mentioned is found in the brain of patients with Alzheimer's disease.

GENERAL BENEFITS

In a review study low concentration of DHEA in elderly men was found to be associated with an increased risk of dying. Other properties of DHEA include its ability to reduce the appetite particularly for fats, to help people lose excess weight and to improve the tone of the skin. In fact, DHEA together with other hormones and antioxidants is now being used in cream form to help reduce the visible effects of skin ageing.

Dosage

The best way to take DHEA is as tablets, in a micronized form so that the active ingredient is easily absorbed in the gut. DHEA in the sulphate form – a much cheaper form to produce than the micronized one – may not be that useful to the tissues because it is not easily assimilated within the body. It can be used in capsule or tablet form, in skin patches, and even under the tongue for easier absorption.

The recommended dose for the micronized form is 25 mg–50 mg daily and for the 7-keto variety is 12.5 mg–25 mg daily.

Women should not use high doses of DHEA because they are able to metabolize, or make use of, any artificially taken DHEA much more easily than men. This means that when a woman takes DHEA, it is easily turned into the different inter-mediaries, including the male hormone testosterone which produces bad side effects. High levels of testosterone in women can cause acne, growth of hair on the face and deep-ening of the voice. Not an attractive possibility by anyone's standards. For fear of these side effects scientists recommend that women should use a reduced dose, perhaps 15 mg–25 mg a day, or use the 7-keto form which does not easily turn into testosterone.

Having said that, there are studies which examined such high doses of DHEA as an extravagant 1600 mg–2000 mg daily, and found that they improved muscle tissue and reduced body fat without any significant side effects. These high doses may be relevant for people who have specific diseases and are under expert medical supervision. There is no obvious reason why healthy people should take anywhere near those high amounts.

The long-term use of low strength hormones has been supported by some experts – even by those opposed to the general idea of anti-ageing medicine – as possibly an effective way of treating some of the signs of ageing.

Side Effects

It has been estimated that the natural, youthful production of DHEA by the body averages 25 mg a day, and this has been used as a guideline for adjusting the dose in tablet form. Taking anything over 50 mg a day increases the risk of side effects. Menstrual bleeding may return in some post-menopausal women, but the bleeding is usually light. Also, taking continuous high doses may make the adrenal glands switch off and stop producing whatever small amounts of natural DHEA they are still capable of.

A Double Warning

Some users have reported severe depression after taking even two or three doses of DHEA but, fortunately, this improved after stopping the treatment. Changing from ordinary DHEA to the 7-keto form did not cause any further depression in these users.

Men with prostate problems should not take DHEA, or at least take it only under close medical supervision. This is because it may increase the prostatic specific antigen (PSA), which indicates an increased risk of prostate cancer.

DHEA is a restricted substance and, in some countries, needs a doctor's prescription. Having said that, there are suppliers who make it available for personal use only in certain instances. Regulations change all the time and it is best to check with your doctor for your particular requirements.

Currently, the use of DHEA in the UK is under the control of the Home Office.

I know of several people who take DHEA whenever they remember, or use it in high doses which cause side effects. Taking DHEA is a serious business and, legal regulations apart, its clinical effects need to be evaluated by a knowledgeable physician. The correct dose for each individual needs to be monitored with regular blood or saliva tests. Usually, it is not necessary to do a test before the treatment starts because it is almost certain that the levels will be below normal. Most people start taking the treatment and do a test about three to six weeks afterwards when the dose can be adjusted, depending on the result.

To summarize with regard to DHEA, it has quite strong advantages but may cause side effects, particularly at high doses. The scientific evidence supporting it is good and growing. It must be taken under medical supervision.

Melatonin

Some people also take melatonin supplements, either on its own or together with DHEA. Melatonin levels also decrease with age and taking it in supplement form is therefore thought to have an impact on age-related problems. A combination of melatonin and DHEA is believed to work more efficiently, improving the chances of fighting age-related changes.

Melatonin is widely used for jet lag and also to improve irregular sleep patterns, so it may be useful for older people who usually have disturbed sleep. It is also a restricted substance in the UK and in some other countries, but it can be obtained with a doctor's prescription.

The anti-ageing benefits of melatonin have only recently been studied in humans. The great majority of research has only been done on mice and on other laboratory animals. One of the main proponents of melatonin is the Italian Professor W. Pierpaoli. At an anti-ageing conference, we discussed his latest research, which shows that post-menopausal women treated with melatonin experience an improvement in their symptoms, together with an improvement of their thyroid levels. The thyroid hormones normally fall with age, and it appears that melatonin has at least a partial beneficial effect in reversing this situation.

I mention this to remind you that hormones work together, and any intake of one hormone may affect the performance of another. This is the basis of the hormonal deregulation theory of ageing which says that, with age, our glands become less able to produce and utilize hormones and, as a result, certain age-related conditions become more pronounced. To counteract this imbalance, and to help the hormones work together again, hormonal supplements and receptor re-sensitizers are used. Remember that carnosine has some receptor re-sensitizing properties, which means that it may facilitate the action of individual hormones on the cells.

Growth Hormone

Apart from DHEA, growth hormone is an important component in the anti-ageing process. Although these are two different hormones, their effects and benefits are sometimes similar or overlapping. Trying to explain the effects of growth hormone is bound to be slightly more difficult than discussing DHEA because growth hormone is connected to several other related chemicals, the action of which needs to be explored. Do not be put off by this. When you understand the basics of how growth hormone works, then its actions and possible benefits will become much clearer.

Human Growth Hormone (hGH or simply GH) is also called somatotropin, and it is produced by the pituitary gland in the brain. This gland is a pea-size organ which also produces several other hormones such as TSH (thyroid stimulating hormone), and sexual hormones which stimulate the production of oestrogen.

As its name suggests, GH is necessary for stimulating normal growth and development in children and for maintaining health in adults. GH is a kind of a 'general construction specialist', needed during everyday activities, such as helping to replace damaged proteins, rebuild cells, replace enzymes and chemical messengers. A lack of growth hormone in childhood can result in stunted growth, and one of the main uses of GH is in treating short stature in children.

The Politics of GH Production

The pituitary gland which produces GH does not work independently, but is under the influence of other regulating hormones and factors, produced by other parts of the brain. For example, GH production is under the control of GHRH (Growth Hormone Releasing Hormone). This factor is produced by the hypothalamus, an important organ in the brain which regulates other glands, just like a central command office.

GHRH is, as the initials explain, a hormone which stimulates release of growth hormone. Another chemical, somatostatin, blocks the release of GH, so GHRH and somatostatin are in a constant tug of war, trying to keep GH at steady, normal levels.

Other hormones such as oestrogen and testosterone may influence the secretion of GH. In fact, as I have already mentioned, most, if not all, hormones in your body depend on each other and none work on their own. GH itself can interact with other hormones such as DHEA which is itself a GH stimulant. An increased production of GH helps normalize low thyroid hormonal levels. Melatonin is a possible releaser of GH, and it is possible that that is how melatonin increased thyroid hormone in Professor Pierpaoli's research mentioned in the previous chapter – by releasing GH which increased thyroid hormone. So you can see that hormones are like individual players in an orchestra, all working together to produce and maintain a masterpiece – you.

When the pituitary gland decides to release GH, it does so in short pulses and not all at once. For example, GH is released at the beginning of sleep. In a 24-hour period, young men experience four main pulses of GH release, whereas young women experience more than four. Exercise and nutrition affect the frequency of these bursts – a bout of physical exercise results in a burst of GH release.

Once released, GH does not do all the work itself but works through an active and strong intermediary. This is produced in the liver and is called Insulin Growth Factor 1 (IGF1, also called somatomedin). Measurement of IGF1 in the blood gives a good indication of what GH is up to.

Both GH and its active equivalent IGF1 need to bind to the cell receptors in order to activate the cell. When the quality and quantity of these cell receptors decreases (as in ageing for example), GH or IGF1 will not be able to bind on to the cells, so they will not have any appreciable effect. The binding of GH to a suitable cell receptor is like the use of a key in a custom-made lock. If the lock is damaged, you can have as many keys as you like, but they will not open that particular lock. This is why some scientists say that it is not just a matter of giving extra GH supplements but also a matter of somehow activating the receptors so that the whole system can work in harmony.

So, to summarize:

1. GHRH is produced by the hypothalamus and stimulates the production of GH from the pituitary gland.
2. GH increases IGF1 in the liver.
3. IGF1 binds to cell receptors and activates the cells to work properly.

Any disturbance of this process, at any stage and for whatever reason, causes the problems related to the lack of GH.

What Does it Mean?

Soma	=	body, from the Greek
Somato-tropin	=	a hormone that 'turns' towards (i.e. supports) the body (GH)
Somato-statin	=	a hormone that 'stops' the effects on the body
Somato-medin	=	a hormone that 'mediates' the effects on the body (IGF1)
Somato-pause	=	a pause in the growth of the body

Growth Hormone Deficiency

A deficiency of GH in adults becomes more severe with age and this can occur from the age of 35–40. Normally, GH production peaks during adolescence and then starts to fall. A 60-year-old man may have only one quarter of the GH secretion of a 20-year-old. Older people also have less frequent bursts of GH release, and these bursts are not as powerful and last for a shorter time than those of younger people.

The lack of GH which comes with age is sometimes referred to as 'somatopause'. The most important consequences of low activity GH are:

- a loss of muscle tissue and strength
- an increase of fat, particularly intra abdominal fat (i.e. fat tissues inside the abdomen)
- a thinning of the bones, which may result in, or contribute to, osteoporosis
- a worsening of glucose metabolism by a reduction in the responsiveness of cells to the actions of insulin, which is a hormone responsible for lowering blood glucose.

There are many other age-related changes attributed to dwindling GH activities:

- decreased energy
- a loss of libido and sexual function
- grey, fragile hair and damaged skin – e.g. wrinkles, due to the loss of collagen, the production of which is normally increased by GH; wound healing becoming slow and imperfect.
- a worsening of mental function, with loss of memory, motivation and concentration
- a reduction of the effectiveness of the immune system.

The Replacement of Growth Hormone

It is a scientific fact that replacement therapy with GH can reverse some, if not all, of the above changes or problems. This has been shown to be true in a number of scientific experiments reported in peer-reviewed, prestigious medical journals such as *The New England Journal of Medicine*.

It is quite surprising to come across respected scientists who say that treatment with GH does not reverse the effects of ageing. It does. Older people lose muscle tissue just because they are getting old, but when they have suitable GH treatment their muscle tissue improves – perhaps not to where it was before, but it improves nevertheless. This is a reversal of an age-related change. It may not affect the underlying rate of ageing in that it will not reverse the rate of the biological ageing clock, nor will it slow it down, but it can give an 'aged' person some of the characteristics of a younger person, albeit temporarily.

The problem is that there are many unanswered questions. We do not know for how long GH can safely be taken; what the best way is to take it; how to decide who is suitable to have the treatment; what to do to reduce the cost of treatment and to reduce its side effects; and whether there are any hidden surprises after long-term treatment. Whatever the answers to these questions may turn out to be, the physiological benefits of GH treatment are now well recognized.

For example, GH makes muscle cells stronger and healthier by increasing their uptake of amino acids. This anabolic effect has raised a glimmer of hope in people who have muscle-wasting diseases, or other myopathies.

GH helps to restore the wall of the bowel to a more youthful state. The lining of the bowel wall progressively becomes thinner with age, causing problems with the normal absorption of food. GH helps prevent this problem by increasing the thickness of the bowel lining. It could be possible to involve carnosine in this as an intermediary. A carnosine–zinc combination was shown to be effective in stimulating the production of IGF1 in the stomach and in the bowel. This increases the number of protective cells in the stomach, and so reduces the damage caused during ulcer formation.

According to supporters of GH treatment, almost all age-related devastation may be improved and repaired following GH replacement. People on GH treatment report sharper vision, better exercise capacity, lower blood pressure, improved memory and a robust libido. Their skin texture improves, and age-related thinning of the skin is reversed. Wound healing and immunity also improve, which is why GH is sometimes used in debilitated patients after surgery.

GH works together with such antioxidants as carnosine or Q10 to soak up free radicals. It creates special chemicals called 'protease inhibitors' which prevent free radicals from further attacking the cells. Even after free radical injury has occurred, GH provides the necessary stimulation for repairing the damaged parts of the cell.

Formal prescribing regulations do not approve the use of GH for anything other than the treatment of stunted stature in children or of those adults who have a definite deficiency of GH resulting in a specific disease. GH is not licensed for use in normal ageing, although the regulations are not clear. According to the exact interpretation of the regulation, all middle-aged and older adults have low levels of GH and IGF1, resulting in specific diseases irrespective of the fact that they are age-related diseases, so GH therapy should, in theory, be available for them.

Artificial Growth Hormone

Modern GH is made synthetically in the laboratory through genetic manipulation. Previously, good quality GH was obtained from the brains of cadavers which was fraught with dangers as it could transmit CJD (Creutzfeldt-Jakob Disease), the human equivalent of BSE or mad cow disease. So, in this respect, the natural form of GH is greatly inferior to a synthetic form.

One of the problems of synthetic GH is that it has to be given by injection. It is also a very expensive treatment. Some doctors also believe that any benefits gained from using injectable GH may decrease with time because too much artificial GH may actually interfere with the normal function of the cell receptors and, as a result, become unable to access the inside of the cell. So it is best to use low, near-physiological doses during treatment. 'Too much' is not necessarily 'better'.

A Regime of Growth Hormone Injections

The injections need to be given daily – sometimes several times a day – following blood tests to evaluate IGF1. A dose of four to eight units a week is considered sufficiently low and free from significant side effects. The results may become apparent after six to ten months of treatment. Follow-up testing is necessary, to keep an eye on the level of IGF1, as well as on the PSA (prostate specific antigen) in men in order to monitor any possible adverse effects on the prostate.

Any side effects from this injection treatment depend on the dose used. Use a high dose of GH and you increase the risk of side effects. Lower the dose and the side effects become less noticeable. Common problems (when the dose is too high) are:

- carpal tunnel syndrome with increased tissue swelling which compresses the nerve at the wrist causing wrist pain
- an increased tendency to diabetes. Diabetic patients, in particular, should only use GH under expert medical supervision, if at all.
- gynecomastia (breast enlargement in both males and females)

- fluid retention
- high blood pressure
- acromegaly (enlargement of the extremities)
- deepening of the voice

Recent experiments also suggest that increased GH may worsen the risk of cancer of the colon, and some doctors believe that high and prolonged use of GH may actually accelerate ageing. So, there you have it. It is all a question of balance.

Secretagogues

Fear of side effects, the enormous costs of treatment, and drug licensing regulations have directed interest to investigating other ways of boosting GH within the body without giving artificial growth hormone shots. It turns out that there are a multitude of substances, both synthetic and natural, which can stimulate the secretion of GH by the pituitary gland.

These substances are called GH secretagogues – a secretagogue being a substance that stimulates a gland to produce another substance. GH secretagogues, rightly or wrongly, are currently very fashionable in the field of anti-ageing therapy. There are new products being announced almost daily and it is extremely difficult to be sure which are effective and which are useless.

Theoretically, all of the benefits of injectable GH are also possible with GH secretagogues, although some people say that secretagogues are even better. Proponents of the use of secretagogues maintain that the pituitary is perfectly able to produce and secrete GH, but that it stops doing so because it receives conflicting orders from higher up in the brain – for example from the hypothalamus, which tells the pituitary what to do via the stimulating agent GHRH. For some reason GHRH fails with age and so it does not stimulate the pituitary to secrete GH. Secretagogues aim to remediate this by remotivating the different parts of the brain which are involved in GH production.

It is generally believed that endurance exercise is one of the best natural ways to increase GH production. However the effects of exercise on GH in older people have not been studied in detail. One particular study did not find any increase in GH or IGF1 after a six-month exercise programme in older people. So, in order to be on the safe side, many people decide to use chemicals in tablet form to increase their GH.

Until recently, it was not very clear whether these secretagogues acted directly on the pituitary and stimulated it to produce GH, or they acted indirectly on the hypothalamus to release GHRH which, in turn, stimulated GH production. In a recent experiment, scientists from Sao Paolo University in Brazil found that at least some of these secretagogues do indeed act directly on the pituitary receptors to stimulate GH release. This is important because it shows that the pituitary is still capable of producing GH and can respond to any signal sent either directly to it, or indirectly through GHRH. Taking secretagogues plus GHRH was shown to have maximum effects in some experimental animal studies. In addition, a few human trials show promising benefits from using this combination.

Pioneering experiments show that there are several sites within the brain tissues which are specifically aimed at binding secretagogues. Secretagogues home in on these sites, bind on to the cells and activate them. Receptors for secretagogues not only exist on the brain but also on other tissues, for example in the heart. Experiments with the secretagogue called hexarelin show that this molecule can have a direct beneficial effect on the heart, particularly when the treatment is prolonged, which has nothing to do with any GH released from the brain.

New brand-name secretagogues are being launched at an alarming rate. At the last count there were over 150 different products but the following are some of the more established.

Growth Hormone Releasing Peptide 6 (GHRP-6), a sequence of six amino acids, is the first synthetic secretagogue (hexarelin). It is one of the most well studied secretagogues but research results are conflicting. It was given to patients for a period of 16 weeks, in a study performed by researchers from the University of Manchester in the United Kingdom. The researchers concluded that hexarelin had no significant beneficial effects on muscle, fat content or bone strength. Taking hexarelin for a long period may also reduce those few benefits experienced originally, as the pituitary gets tired of the continuous stimulation and finally gives up. Whether this effect, called attenuation, is seen with other secretagogues is not clear but it is possible.

Other experiments show that GHRP-6 stimulates the release of GH in cycles which are similar to natural GH release cycles. Several experiments show some positive results from GHRP-6 use. In recent experiments, hexarelin-related compounds were shown to be effective in inducing penile erection in rats, if given by injection in the brain. This could be awkward if it proves to have the same effects in humans. Brain injections for impotence!

Symbiotropin (ProHGH) contains amino acid sequences, as well as plant-derived L-dopa and other plant chemicals which are said to regulate IGF1. It is thought to be effective in stimulating the pituitary through GHRH to secrete GH in pulses and thus mimics the natural pattern of GH release.

Meditropin is a stronger and more modern variant of the above, and is currently only available on a doctor's prescription. It contains symbiotropin and GHRH co-factors.

Ghrelin is a series of 28 amino acids formed in the stomach, so it is a natural variant. It is a strong GH releaser which works by binding to GH receptors and stimulating its effective release.

Somatomed, a secretagogue produced by Vespro Ltd., was found to be useful in chronic fatigue syndrome (CFS).

Evaluation following the treatment of 200 patients suffering from CFS, showed that significant numbers of them experienced improvement in sleep patterns, better cognition, a decrease in muscle pain and fatigue. Side effects of this treatment were transient muscle pain and mild swelling of the hands and feet.

GHRH analogues or stimulants. An experimental GHRH-analogue – i.e. a chemical having a similar structure to the original GHRH – has been found to be effective, and its actions persisted after long-term treatment. Among the advantages of the treatment were increasing IGF1 levels and many clinical improvements such as increased skin thickness, lean body mass and improved libido.

Other experimental secretagogues are so new that they have not even got proper names yet and are known only by their laboratory codes. For example, the one called NN703, is given by mouth and has similar effects to those of GHRP-6, as above. Another one called MK677 was found to have positive benefits on the bone, particularly helping to increase bone mass in the hip joint and to reduce the risk of osteoporosis.

Some secretagogues are enclosed in liposomes – minute special fat globules which can penetrate the skin and release any active substance they are carrying – for better absorption and can be given by oral spray. Individual substances which increase GH production, and many of these are included in the secretagogue combinations discussed above, are:

- the amino acid glutamine which increases GH secretion by 15%
- L-dopa, a drug used in Parkinson's disease, is effective in men over 60 years old
- the amino acids arginine, lysine, and ornithine (usually at high doses of 2 g daily)
- minerals such as potassium, zinc, magnesium, calcium, chromium and vanadium
- GABA, a type of amino acid
- homeopathic preparations of GH which are claimed to be able to stimulate GH release
- carnosine, possibly. It modulates the activity of the minerals zinc, magnesium, chromium and vanadium, which are thought to play a role in GH release. Also, although not yet proven, it is theoretically possible that carnosine is able to increase the sensitivity of the hypothalamus through special proteins and so protect and/or repair the receptors. If that is the case, carnosine would act as a 'hypothalamic and pituitary re-sensitizer', suitable for indirectly reactivating hormonal secretion by these two organs. There have been some animal experiments pointing us in the right direction. For example, it is known that carnosine modulates the NMDA receptor in the brain, and regulates the actions of nitric oxide (NO) which, in turn, balances GH secretion. Incidentally, that is why the amino acid arginine is a good GH releaser, because it stimulates the production of NO.

Other Releasers of GH

The Australian yeast extract Vegemite, similar to Marmite in the UK, was found to be a good GH releaser. These yeast extracts are effective in increasing GH production by about 30%, which is the average increase experienced from some of the synthetic secretagogues. There is anecdotal evidence that drinks such as Newcastle Brown Ale are potentially able to increase GH but the exact mechanism of this is still not clear.

The drug GHB (gamma hydroxy butyrate) has been proven to have a strong releasing effect on GH, being able to cause an amazing 600% increase in GH secretion. GHB is, however, banned in several countries because it has the potential to be abused as a 'date rape' drug. Incidentally, GHB is believed by some doctors to be one of the best anti-ageing drugs available, if used properly.

Synthetic GH versus Secretagogues

GH is a promising anti-ageing treatment, but how to get it into the body is another matter. Artificial GH given by injection produces a 500–600% increase of GH in the body, but the treatment is expensive and has the potential for side effects. There is research showing that synthetic GH can be given not only by injection but also in nasal spray form or in patches, although more research is needed to support this.

Using secretagogues is also costly, and it may increase GH by only 30% but it is also less liable to cause side effects. People who choose to use secretagogues should make sure that the preparation they are using is at least partly supported by research. Some advertisements make it very confusing and difficult to get the real picture, claiming that a particular product is a real (synthetic or natural) GH molecule, when in fact it is only a poor quality secretagogue.

Certain claims made about secretagogues are completely invalid. Many products are advertized by gimmicky words such as 'revolutionary', 'unique', 'scientifically produced', 'ground-breaking'. The truth is that only some of these products have actually been found to be somewhat effective, and many of the rest are not well studied substances.

Overall, some products may have measurable effects, whereas others may not. Scientific studies of these substances are few and far between, and the few studies that exist do not always show clear benefits. As things stand at the moment, it is a matter of getting as much information about the product as you can and deciding for yourself. If after, say, four to six months you do not experience any obvious benefits, then it may be time to stop using that particular product. As always, you should work together with your medical practitioner to find products which are suitable for you.

The bottom line is that injectable GH should only be used in selected cases under medical supervision. It is expensive and has the potential for side effects. Lower doses are better in the long term. Secretagogues are used by a wide section of the public but consideration should be given to the cost, the medical evidence supporting the particular secretagogue and the fact that there are no guarantees about the results. Remember that GH does not affect the underlying ageing process, but may improve some of the signs of ageing on the body.

Co-enzyme Q10

Over and over again, nature comes up with chemical masterpieces which are deceptively simple but have an astonishing variety of benefits. Carnosine is one such compound, co-enzyme Q10 is another. These ingenious substances are 'pluripotent', in other words they are effective in many different biological processes and have multiple actions.

Co-enzyme Q10, or simply 'Q10', is one of the most abundant nutrients in your body. It is found in almost every tissue, and its description 'ubiquinone' attests to that. Its presence is 'ubiquitous' and, chemically, it belongs to the family of 'quinones'.

Your body soaks up some Q10 from food, but the average Q10 content of the Western diet is estimated at 100 times less than the amount your body actually needs for its everyday activities. Fortunately, your body is able to create new Q10 molecules under its own steam, to top up its supplies. However, this production of brand new Q10 becomes progressively less efficient with age, and here we encounter the old argument as to whether it is necessary to do something about this age-related deficiency, or just go along with nature's plan and leave things as they are. You will see that I support the former point of view and believe that, on balance, it is best to use extra Q10 supplements during ageing.

A Mighty Ally

One of the main jobs of Q10 is to offer antioxidant protection. Q10 is present at the very heart of the metabolism, the mitochondria. It is able to quench any free radicals created by the mitochondria, which burn oxygen during the process of producing energy for fuelling the body. The mitochondria are the energy factories where the transformation of different chemicals produces energy. They utilize a tremendous amount of oxygen and so overproduction of free radicals is inevitable. Trouble is always brewing inside the mitochondria. The presence of Q10 within the mitochondria is nature's way of dealing with these excessive free radicals, which need to be inactivated before they can cause any serious mischief.

Excessive free radical production speeds up the process of apoptosis which results in the death of too many normal cells. As I have explained before, a moderate degree of apoptosis is necessary to get rid of any damaged cells with minimal disruption to the surrounding cells, but an accelerated apoptosis eliminates so many cells that those left behind become unable to cope with their normal duties. This leaves the tissues in shambles. Q10, being 50 times stronger than vitamin E, protects against this extreme cell death by reducing the cell exposure to free radicals.

Your mitochondria come furnished with their own special DNA supply which needs to be protected as efficiently as the rest of your DNA. Normally, the DNA molecule in the central nucleus of the cells is relatively well protected against the rigours of ageing, but the DNA which is inside the mitochondria is exposed to an immense amount of free radical hits and it is liable to be easily damaged. In fact, many scientists believe that injury to the mitochondrial DNA is one of the first signs seen during the ageing process. Drastic measures are needed here, and Q 10 comes to the rescue.

Several experiments done on mice show that Q10 is able to protect mitochondrial DNA from this kind of damage. The very latest studies report that Q10 supplements may also protect human mitochondrial DNA from free radical attack. This is good news, because damaged DNA can build up over time. This disrupts the normal workings of the mitochondria, causing a 'power meltdown', eventually resulting in ageing and early death.

Co-enzyme Q10 as an Energiser

In addition to its antioxidant activity, Q10 is also very accomplished at boosting overall energy and muscle strength. It facilitates the production of chemical energy from the burning of oxygen inside the mitochondria. Scientists who studied the effects of Q10 on rats, found that it can protect the animals' capacity to respond to stress and improves their muscle endurance.

When experimenting with heart tissue from people with heart disease, scientists discovered that young cells normally recover much faster than older cells following stress, such as the lack of oxygen. However, when these cells were pre-treated with Q10, the difference between young and old was abolished, and the older cells recovered as quickly as the young ones. Amazing isn't it! This shows that Q10 may have a role to play in maintaining the muscle metabolism in older people when the blood supply is interrupted, during a heart attack, for example.

Q10 and Heart Disease

The concentration of Q10 in the heart muscle plummets with age, and is usually lower in patients who have heart disease than in those of similar age without any heart problems. Several properly performed scientific trials have shown that Q10 is effective in reducing some of the symptoms of stroke, heart failure, heart attack and angina.

It works like this. The 'bad' fat, LDL (low density lipo-protein), carries cholesterol around the body via the bloodstream. Free radical damage to LDL is an important cause of atherosclerosis, which is thickening of the arteries and may result in heart problems and stroke. Vitamin E and Q10 are the antioxidants which play a serious part in reducing the union between free radicals and LDL within the blood vessels and so reduce the risk of atherosclerosis. Studies performed both in animals and in humans have proved that Q10 is particularly useful in this situation and that it can be used to prevent heart disease in the long term.

Other experiments show that taking 150 mg of Q10 a day is effective at slashing the frequency of angina pain almost by half. Also, if Q10 is given to patients who undergo a heart operation, it considerably reduces the amount of injury to the heart muscle, both during and after the operation.

Vitamin E – Friend or Foe?

The use of vitamin E on its own may, for some strange reason, worsen free radical attack on LDL on certain occasions. This process is called 'tocopherol-mediated peroxidation' – remember that vitamin E is also called tocopherol. In this case, vitamin E behaves not as an anti-oxidant, but as a pro-oxidant. The presence of Q10 though, protects against this worrying phenomenon and turns vitamin E back to behave as an anti-oxidant again.

So, vitamin E and Q10 need to be taken together, ideally in a single combination tablet, for maximum protection against lipid peroxidation. Experiments confirm that Q10 plus vitamin E is a more effective strategy against atherosclerosis than Q10 or vitamin E given separately.

As you probably remember from chapter 1, the chemical nitric oxide (NO) if left unbalanced may play a significant role during inflammation which may well contribute to atherosclerosis. A toxic by-product of nitric oxide called 'peroxynitrite', can be kept at bay by using Q10 supplements. Patients who were treated with a daily dose of 150 mg of Q10 for five days, had a decreased amount of peroxynitrite in their blood which means that their risk of developing athero-sclerosis and, consequently, heart problems, was reduced.

This was confirmed by another experiment using animal brain tissue, which showed that both NO and our old friend MDA (malondialdehyde) are kept low after toxic injury, but only if the brain is treated with very large doses of Q10. The benefits shown in animal experiments have also been confirmed during human clinical trials. Several studies using relatively high doses of Q10 (150 mg–600 mg) showed that heart disease patients may experience an improvement in their angina, with an ability to walk further than usual and a reduced need for medication.

In some of these trials, the blood levels of other anti-oxidants (such as vitamin E and vitamin C) were increased as if by magic, even though Q10 was the only nutrient supplied. This means that Q10 may have the ability to fuel the produc-tion of other antioxidants in the body.

Apart from its use in reducing the symptoms of angina, Q10 is also useful in rectifying heart failure, and several experiments support this. Heart failure patients may experi-ence many symptoms including:

- shortness of breath
- swelling of the legs

- tiredness
- blue or pale extremities
- loss of appetite

I am not, of course, suggesting that Q10 can make these symptoms disappear completely but it may improve the overall condition, particularly when taken in association with conventional drugs.

Patients who use cholesterol-lowering drugs called statins, may benefit from Q10 supplements, because it is believed that some of these statin drugs block the actions of Q10. When Q10 is given as an additional supplement, however, the statins and Q10 work together to lower cholesterol even further. Having said that, trials with the cholesterol-lowering drugs called 'pravastatin' and 'atorvastatin' have shown that these two do not always decrease Q10, so people who take these two particular drugs may not need to take additional Q10 supplements. Atorvastatin has, in fact, been withdrawn in some countries due to fears that it may cause muscle problems.

New studies also show that Q10 reduces abnormally high blood pressure. In a typical study, 59 patients with high blood pressure were given either 120 mg of Q10 or a placebo for two months. The Q10 group experienced a fall in blood pressure, and a decrease of LDL, together with an increase in the 'good' fat HDL. Q10 was also able to reduce blood glucose and improve the ability of insulin to deal with glucose more effectively. This is good news because, as I have already explained, too much glucose in the blood contributes to glycosylation and AGE formation.

> **Case Study**
> The benefits of Q10 in limiting brain damage after the oxygen supply is cut off, are well known. This makes it a promising supplement to use in stroke. In a discussion about the anti-stroke benefits of Q10, I was told of a woman who was taking 400 mg of Q10 a day when she had a head injury resulting in a stroke. She was in coma and was expected to die within a few days, but she recovered after ten days. Was this because her brain was protected by the Q10? Maybe. Other similar unsubstantiated cases have also been reported.

Macular Degeneration

This age-related condition is one of the most common causes of partial blindness in the world. It is thought to be, at least in part, due to free radicals attacking the retina at the back of the eye.

In a very recent study, Italian scientists measured the Q10 content of the blood in patients with macular degeneration and found it to be lower than that of healthy people of the same age. Patients with macular degeneration were also less able to deal with free radicals than healthy people. The researchers concluded that Q10 supplements may well protect against macular degeneration.

Cancer

Unconfirmed experiments show that Q10 may be effective in reducing the advance of cancers, such as those of the prostate and breast. The concentration of Q10 in the blood of people suffering from prostate or breast cancer is low anyway, but giving high doses of Q10 to such patients reduces some of the effects of these cancers. For example, it lowers the level of PSA in prostate cancer, high PSA or prostatic specific antigen being a general sign that cancer of the prostate is a possibility. But these are small trials and larger ones are needed. If this anti-cancer potential of Q10 proves to be case, then Q10 will be an ideal partner to use with DHEA which may, in some instances, worsen the risk of prostate or breast cancer.

Although Q10 was found to protect the heart during certain types of chemotherapy for cancer, particularly if used in association with vitamin E, its widespread use during chemotherapy is not generally recommended, in case it worsens free radical activity during the treatment. Again, more research is needed to clarify this.

Brain Health

Q10 treatment helps improve brain function. This is achieved in a variety of ways:

- It protects against free radicals which are massing to unleash their power onto the brain cells. If left uncontrolled, this destruction could result in the production of beta amyloid which is found in the brain of Alzheimer's disease patients.
- It limits overproduction of glutamate which may cause excitotoxicity, the brain injury caused by too much stimulation.
- Q10 improves the general metabolism of brain cells.

Some patients with Parkinson's disease have a low Q10 concentration in their brains. This, some scientists speculate, suggests that Q10 supplements may help lessen some of the symptoms of the disease.

Gum Health

Q10 is used by some people in oral spray form to prevent and treat gum disease. It reduces gum bleeding and helps maintain healthy gum tissues. Gum disease is one of the commonest problems related to ageing, and it is this that causes the loss of teeth. Japanese researchers found that Q10 reduces swelling and pain of the gums. Some people apply the oil from Q10 capsules directly on to their gums, but the spray for direct application on the gums, or the tablets taken by mouth are also effective.

General Energy and Muscular Conditions

Many of my patients who take Q10 supplements experience an increase in their levels of energy. This makes them more active and reduces feelings of tiredness. Q10 is also used to fight several conditions which cause muscle weakness such as muscular dystrophy, multiple sclerosis, and other myopathies because it improves energy in the muscle and protects the mitochondria. However, sufferers from these conditions are generally advised by their practitioner to take Q10 in higher doses than usual.

You will remember that growth hormone or DHEA are also used by some sufferers of muscular conditions. Combining Q10 with growth hormone or with DHEA may bestow stronger benefits on some of these patients.

A Skin Rejuvenator

The health-supporting properties of Q10 make it a convenient substance for the cosmetic industry to use. Creams containing Q10 are marketed as being effective in reducing the results of skin ageing. Q10 is used with other products for maximum anti-ageing support to the skin. Examples of these are:

- aloe vera
- antioxidants
- retinol
- DHEA/melatonin complexes

How to Take Co-ezyme Q10

Q10 needs to be taken with some form of fat, because its absorption is enhanced in the presence of fat in the diet. There are capsules containing Q10 mixed with oil and these are thought to be more suitable than simple tablets. It is important to choose good quality Q10 which means that it has to be of the expensive pharmaceutical grade quality, and standardized to provide equal amounts of Q10 with every capsule.

I have already mentioned that it is best to take it together with vitamin E, and many preparations do indeed contain this vitamin within the same capsule as the Q10. The available preparations come in different strengths, commonly 10 mg, 30 mg and 100 mg. Most people who take 30 mg of Q10 are adequately covered but there are others who take higher doses without any side effects.

Idebenone

This is a close variant of Q10, which is claimed to possess a wider range of benefits than Q10 itself. It is stronger than Q10 and affords a better protection against free radicals. It is a generally more efficient chemical than Q10.

Its antioxidant actions have aroused interest in the treatment of brain problems such as dementia. In a German trial, a six month course of 90 mg of Idebenone a day was found to create a significant improvement in patients with Alzheimer's disease. It improved memory, attention span, and orientation and it slowed down the natural progression of Alzheimer's, albeit temporarily. This is because it offers protection to the membrane of the nerve cells, enhances the speed of information transmission, and powers up the brain metabolism. It encourages the production of nerve growth factors which are needed for the normal grooming of the nerve cells.

Some people recommend taking both Q10 and Idebenone for maximum benefits. Side effects are mild nausea, anxiety and sleep difficulties. Remember that both Q10 and Idebenone are energy-boosters and increase general metabolism. The normal dose is 45 mg once or twice a day, but double this amount can be used for specific diseases. Idebenone can be taken with a wide variety of other anti-ageing drugs for best effects.

The bottom line is that Q10 is cheap and easily available. Its actions are multiple and a good deal of the research is positive. It is becoming increasingly accepted by medical practitioners in general. Do remember that it is best taken together with vitamin E and other antioxidants.

Methylation Enhancers

Without methylation you will die in a matter of days. Defective methylation is a time bomb, and the biological clock of those who cannot repair this deficiency is about to run down.

Faulty methylation causes several problems, but one of the most important is the increase of homocysteine which worsens the risk of developing a number of age-related diseases. Homocysteine is a type of amino acid, a by-product of another amino acid, methionine. Whereas methionine is essential to your health, as it takes part in many normal processes, homocysteine is exactly the opposite, having been associated with illness, as we shall see below.

The Streaker's Cycle

Homocysteine is methionine without its clothes on, a kind of streaker causing disruption during the game of life. It is what remains when good methionine is used by the tissues to methylate your proteins and DNA. Normally, as soon as homocysteine is formed, it is quickly clothed with methyl groups and converted back to methionine again.

Folic acid, vitamins of the B group and the chemical SAMe (see below) are needed for this conversion to take place. They are the police officers and the clothes-bearers who cover homocysteine up quickly, before disorder can become unmanageable. Homocysteine can also be transformed through several steps into a very useful antioxidant, glutathione, again with the help of vitamins of the B group. This cycle continues over and over again throughout life.

If, for any reason, any of the steps of this cycle are disturbed, then homocysteine cannot adequately revert to useful methionine or even to glutathione, and so it remains behind ready to cause trouble. I do not know if you have ever been into a stadium with several streakers running loose for hours. I have not, but I can imagine what happens. Everything must end in total chaos.

One reason for the defective operation of the methionine–homocysteine cycle is lack of folic acid and a deficiency of vitamins of the B group, such as vitamin B6 and B12. When these vitamins are low in your tissues, the homocysteine cycle misfires and becomes unable to operate at full speed. Too much homocysteine is created but it cannot be quickly covered up and inactivated.

The problem is that these vitamins become progressively less effective with age, even in healthy older people. It is as if these molecular policemen become too sluggish to run after the streakers. In addition, any deficiency of these vitamins in your diet will make matters worse, the equivalent of not supplying enough police officers or clothes during the game. Consuming folic acid and B vitamins is essential in keeping the cycle of homocysteine going. These vitamins should be obtained mainly from green vegetables and fruit. The mineral zinc is also used somewhere in this process, to make matters a bit easier. It is a kind of a policeman's hat which covers the sensitive parts of the streaker until further help arrives. Zinc is obtained from oysters, pulses, wholegrain cereals and lean beef which, as we have seen, is also a good source of carnosine.

Why, you may ask, is it necessary for 'nice' methionine to be transformed to noxious homocysteine in the first place? The answer is that methionine is needed to methylate other essential molecules down the line, such as proteins, enzymes, DNA, phospholipids and so on. During this process, methionine creates methyl groups which are picked up by carrier chemicals such as SAMe, and then taken to those constituents of your body which consume methyl groups for their own maintenance.

Homocysteine is a necessary by-product of this process, and it is meant to be inactivated quickly thereafter. But, as we have seen, things do not always work as smoothly, and homocysteine can stay behind. High levels of homocysteine mean that the methylation processes in the body are below par. The body is able to deal with defective methylation for a short while, but not for long.

Heart Disease

Health conditions which are thought to be aggravated by high homocysteine include heart disease and stroke. There are several reasons for this:

- homocysteine encourages the clumping together of platelets resulting in abnormal clotting of blood.

- It makes it more difficult for the arteries to relax as it interferes with nitric oxide which normally keeps the blood vessels nice and wide, and therefore causes obstruction of the normal blood flow.

- In the mitochondria of the heart muscle cells, homocysteine interacts with iron and copper metal ions to speed up production of free radicals. These, in turn, encourage 'bad' fat LDL to cause even more oxidation-related damage.

Eventually, heart attack, stroke and other circulation problems, such as thrombosis of the legs and lungs, become more likely. Problems related to high homocysteine are particularly likely to happen in people aged 50 and over, perhaps due to the fact that the nutrients which limit homocysteine, such as vitamin B, become less abundant with age. High homocysteine is considered by doctors to be a risk factor for heart disease, equally as important as other heart disease risk factors such as smoking, lack of exercise and obesity.

Dementia

There are concerns that high homocysteine in the blood plays a part in causing Alzheimer's disease. Alzheimer's disease patients have low levels of folic acid in their brain, which may be a sign that the homocysteine cycle is blocked. A Swedish study of 370 people aged over 75 years, found that those with low levels of folic acid and vitamin B12 were at an increased risk of developing Alzheimer's. At the same time, those who had high levels of these two vitamins were at a low risk.

The chemical SAMe which helps reduce the amounts of homocysteine, is usually low in the brain of Alzheimer's disease patients. Homocysteine can also damage the lining of the nerves and this is seen particularly in patients who have diabetes.

Liver Disease

Researchers trying to clarify the actions of homocysteine have shown that this chemical can cause liver problems. This could be due to the pro-oxidant activity of homocysteine as it helps create free radicals which attack the liver cells.

Homocysteine also interferes with the liver enzymes. Alcohol causes liver damage and, apart from the toxic effects of alcohol directly on to the liver cells, this damage is also explained by the fact that alcohol reduces the amounts of B vitamins in the liver.

Depression

High homocysteine has been associated with depression. This is because the chemical serotonin, which reduces the symptoms of depression, needs to be constantly methylated in order to keep up its good work. Slow methylation results in inactive serotonin which cannot work properly in the brain, resulting in depression. A sign of low methylation is high homocysteine.

You will see below that chemicals such as SAMe which encourage methylation may improve serotonin levels which, in turn, decrease depression, as well as reduce homocysteine. You can see here how one chemical affects another, just like hormones which affect one another. Deficiency of one chemical causes repercussions right through the entire system.

Ageing

The ageing process itself may be affected by homocysteine. The telomeres (the end parts of the DNA molecule) are usually damaged by free radicals and start shrinking with age. Short telomeres are one of the signs of ageing. It was found that homocysteine accelerates this process of telomere destruction. The exact explanation why this happens is not very clear at present, but it implies that nutrients which reduce homocysteine may well have a protective effect on telomeres.

How to Deal with Homocysteine

So far I have mentioned some of the problems encountered when there are high homocysteine levels. But what can you do about all of this? Is there a way to help yourself?

It is possible to have blood tests for homocysteine and to assess whether you are at risk. The higher the value of homocysteine, the higher the risk of disease. The good news is that homocysteine can be reduced, and that methylation can be increased by simple changes in your diet and by taking the right supplements. The best diet to reduce homocysteine is a combination diet containing:

- low fat dairy products
- fruits and vegetables
- fish
- dry cereals, not those soaked in water or milk
- small quantities of lean pork and beef.

Factors and chemicals which adjust and modulate methylation are used by many millions of people across the world. Two main examples of these, apart from vitamins of the B group, are SAMe and TMG.

SAMe

In my book *Stay Young Longer – Naturally* (Vega Publishers, 2001) I considered SAMe to be one of the essential ingredients of the 'elixir of youth'. I still do. SAMe stands for

S-Adenosyl-Methionine and it is a natural chemical found in all living cells. It is a result of the union between the amino acid methionine and the energy chemical ATP (adenosine triphosphate). SAMe plays a serious part in promoting healthy methylation, as well as helping the body to produce sufficient quantities of the antioxidant glutathione and hence reduce the overall concentration of homocysteine.

Any reduction of the vitamins B6, B12 and of folic acid disrupts the normal metabolism of SAMe and therefore may increase homocysteine and reduce useful glutathione. Conditions that may reduce the normal amounts of SAMe in the body include:

- dementia
- liver disease
- depression
- alcoholism
- the ageing process in general.

It is not exactly known whether these conditions are the cause or the result of low SAMe, but research will clarify this point in the next few years. Whatever the situation, these conditions are irrevocably associated with high homocysteine and anything that lowers homocysteine also improves SAMe. Most of the actions of SAMe are the exact opposites of the actions of homocysteine.

SAMe and Depression

Many doctors practising alternative medicine say that SAMe is one of the most effective and safe antidepressants available. Clinical trials have found that SAMe is as effective in relieving depression as the prescription-only antidepressant imipramine, and it does not have its side effects. The antidepressant actions of SAMe have also been studied in comparison with other prescription antidepressants and found to be equal or superior in many cases.

SAMe versus Herbs

SAMe is sometimes compared to herbal antidepressants or brain nutrients such as:

- St John's wort
- kava kava
- ginseng
- ginkgo biloba

However, SAMe is even more natural than herbal antidepressants. Herbal chemicals are obviously not as natural for humans as they are for plants. It is more natural for people to use something like SAMe which is found in all human cells, in preference to something that is found only in plants.

SAMe is also suitable for treating depression resulting from illnesses such as alcoholism, fibromyalgia and chronic arthritis. It is useful not only in curing the actual condition but also in relieving the depression which is caused as a result of that condition. SAMe helps increase the brain chemical serotonin which, as I have mentioned, is responsible for improving the symptoms of depression.

Serotonin helps to keep you awake and active, and it is more efficient during the day. It could be considered the opposite of melatonin which is useful for inducing sleep and which works during the night. SAMe is needed to adjust this balance between serotonin and melatonin and therefore it helps maintain a healthy sleeping–waking cycle.

The way SAMe works is by helping serotonin bind easily to the cell receptors. It also improves the function of the cell membrane by increasing production of phosphatidyl choline, one of its essential constituents. SAMe is one of the most important methylating agents in the brain. Loss of brain methylation has not only been blamed for depression but is also associated with ageing in general.

The Liver

SAMe helps protect the liver against alcohol and other toxic damage. Drugs which destroy the liver cells include oestrogens, anti-inflammatories and painkillers, but SAMe shields the liver against these. Supplements which support the actions of SAMe in the liver are silymarin, vitamin E and lipoic acid.

Arthritis

Some patients suffering from joint problems and arthritis have been using SAMe with good results. In experiments it was found to improve the structure of the cartilage and thus relieve some of the problems related to osteoarthritis.

As long ago as 1987 over 22,000 patients took part in clinical trials evaluating the benefits of SAMe in arthritis, so it is a relatively well studied remedy. It is used by people who have other forms of arthritis such as rheumatoid arthritis, as well as by those with fibromyalgia, osteoporosis and joint injuries. As opposed to certain anti-inflammatories, SAMe is able to protect the lining of the stomach against acid injury, whereas some anti-inflammatories may actually damage the lining of the stomach. It can be used in association with the anti-arthritis nutrients chondroitin and glucosamine for joint support.

Dose

Dosage depends on the problems being treated.

- Higher doses are usually needed in depression – 200 mg–400 mg twice a day initially and then increasing to three or four times a day.
- Similar or even higher strengths are used for patients with liver problems and arthritis. People usually start with a low dose and increase it as necessary.
- For general anti-ageing and methylation support the average dose is 200 mg–400 mg once or twice daily.

SAMe is quite expensive in the long term but costs are expected to fall when better ways of manufacturing it are found. Taking extra supplements of a cheaper chemical called TMG (see below) may reduce the necessity for taking the full dose of SAMe which brings the cost down appreciably. TMG and SAMe work together, complementing each other. The 'enteric coated' tablets are manufactured specifically for better absorption and they should not be cut in half, nor should they be exposed to sunlight.

Side effects are rare, but include occasional nausea and stomach upset. The side effects are generally well tolerated and improve after a while. In one experiment SAMe was proven to be free from significant side effects after two years of continuous use.

In another experiment involving 734 participants, only 10 people had mild side effects due to SAMe whereas 13 people apparently had side effects just by taking the dummy treatment, or placebo. People who suffer from the manic form of depression should not use SAMe because it makes the condition worse.

TMG

Tri-Methyl-Glycine (TMG, also called 'betaine') is another methylating agent. As the name suggests, TMG has three methyl groups which are easily donated to other structures in need of methylation, particularly the DNA. Donating a methyl group to homocysteine, transforms it into the useful amino acid methionine as explained above. In theory, because it can help lower homocysteine, it also reduces the risk of heart attacks and stroke.

Side effects include mild headaches or muscle tension at high doses, but these usually improve after reducing the dose. It comes in 500 mg tablets and in powder form and it should be taken in association with vitamins B6 and B12 to help maintain the methylating cycle of homocysteine.

A Summary of Methylation

Although the workings of the methylation cycle appear convoluted, in reality they are not. Several illnesses which are related to methylation become more likely when methylation is slow, and may improve when methylation is speeded up. Nutrients such as SAMe, TMG and vitamin B keep this process going and so reduce the likelihood of methylation-dependant diseases.

A sign of how active the methylation processes are in the body is given by homocysteine. If homocysteine is high, it means that methylation is defective. If it is normal, it means that methylation is fine.

SAMe, vitamins of the B group and other methylating nutrients need to be taken both in the diet and in supplements. SAMe can be expensive however. These nutrients help prevent or treat certain age-related illness, but do not, as a rule, appear to reverse the underlying rate of ageing.

Holistic Anti-Ageing Medicine

Taking pills and supplements to try to reduce the signs of ageing is only the beginning. If you want to increase your chances of living a healthy, active life for as long as possible you should also explore other ways of achieving this aim, apart from taking pills.

Regular exercise is one of the most efficient ways of overcoming a number of age-related problems. Remember, however, that too much exercise, lasting over 45 minutes at a time, may actually fuel the production of free radicals and so it should be avoided. The best exercises to keep your body really fit are:

- swimming
- brisk walking
- dancing
- light gym exercises
- aerobics
- gentle weight lifting

● Oriental exercises such as yoga, tai chi and chi kung.

Suitable nutrition should also be high on your agenda. I have discussed anti-ageing nutrition extensively in some of my other books (*Stay Young Longer – Naturally*, and *The Age Defying Cookbook*). Suffice it to say that, due to questions raised about the nutrient content of our modern diet, it is increasingly becoming recognized amongst nutritionists that we need to supplement our diet with extra nutritional supplements in tablet form.

I have mentioned many times that all anti-ageing treatments are a matter of balance. The same is true of our diet. You should try and strike a balance between gorging yourself on foods that you do not like but which are good for you, and having enough freedom to enjoy your life without too many unpleasant restrictions on the food you consume.

In addition to good nutrition and exercise, mental attitudes and positive thinking are also essential in fighting ageing. There is no point in taking a few pills and doing some exercise, when your brain remains neglected, and your thoughts become stale. You need to see growing older as a bonus rather than as a burden. Your aim should be to face ageing straight on but to maintain as many characteristics of youth as possible, and this includes a good, effective brain and a positive mental outlook. I have discussed all of these aspects in detail in previous books but there are other informative books which deal with the matter, such as *Brain Longevity*, (Warner Books, New York, 1997) by Dharma Singh Khalsa.

It is important to realize that nutrition, mental and physical exercises, and anti-ageing medication need to be used together, so we make a continuing effort through our lifestyle to defeat problems related to ageing for as long as possible. You should constantly question the things you do for your health, see if they can be improved and keep an eye on new developments which may help you.

However, do not be fooled by false or sensational advertising or claims. Ask to see the proof behind each product and, if there is no proof that it works, ask yourself whether you want to try it and see, or move on to something else more promising.

Here are two examples to illustrate how effective anti-ageing medication can be in certain aspects of everyday life.

CASE NUMBER 1

Two married couples in their seventies decided to experiment with carnosine. Both couples were doing approximately the same amount of exercise and ate the same kind of diet and followed a similar lifestyle. One member of each couple took 50 mg of carnosine a day for four months whereas their partner did not.

Their party trick was to ask their friends and relatives to guess who was on carnosine and who was not. The funny thing was that most of the time their friends and relatives guessed correctly. This shows you that, no matter what research says, some supplements can indeed have a noticeable impact on whether an individual actually looks healthier or not. Whether the supplement in question truly changes things inside you is a different matter. It may or it may not. How you look, how you feel and what other people think about your appearance is, however, very relevant in life.

CASE NUMBER 2

One of my patients, a woman aged 45 was using over 80 different tablets and capsules a day, as well as doing a lot of exercise trying to keep fit. She considered herself to be very healthy and 'in the know' regarding health matters. However, after undergoing some blood tests and anti-ageing computerized assessments she discovered that her scores were surprisingly bad.

The amount of medication she was taking was not really relevant to ageing, and her exercise regime was excessive. She did not pay any attention to the health of her brain but wanted to remain young at all costs, hating the idea of getting chronologically older.

Following a selective reduction of her medication and a decrease in exercise time, she also underwent a series of counselling sessions to learn how to cope with her increasing age, and to see her own ageing as a natural and healthy part of life. She was of course started on carnosine 100 mg–150 mg a day, as well as DHEA, Q10 and SAMe. After six months of this treatment, her computerized scores improved considerably, and all her detailed blood and urine tests were completely normal.

This highlights one of the most important and frequently neglected aspects of anti-ageing medicine, that it is necessary to use a holistic approach to deal with any problems and not try to deal with problems individually.

Many of the treatments discussed in this book only affect certain aspects of ageing, and questions still remain as to whether other aspects of the ageing process can be stopped completely or even reversed. However, a combination of suitable medication with a healthy lifestyle can go a long way in helping you through the ageing process.

What matters is you. If you feel satisfied with a particular nutrient or drug, if you enjoy your lifestyle and if you are content with your plan of action, then so be it. We only have a comparatively short time on this earth and we should make the most of it. But also remember that you can influence that time, to a certain degree. Choose wisely and you will increase it both in quality and in quantity. It's up to you. Choose poorly, and you will make it even shorter.

Glossary

Alzheimer's dementia – an age-related form of brain damage resulting in severe forgetfulness, inability to look after oneself, cognition problems and disorientation

Antioxidants – substances which reduce or fight free radicals

Apoptosis – the 'falling off' of cells. It is a natural type of orderly and programmed cell death which eliminates damaged cells while leaving healthy cells behind untouched. It is the opposite of 'necrosis' which is a disorderly and widespread cell death.

Atherosclerosis – the thickening of the inside part of the arteries which is in contact with the blood. Fatty deposits, small blood clots and other by-products of inflammation may block the flow of blood.

Cross-over study – half of the participants in the study are given the real treatment to be tested, and the other half are given a placebo. After a certain time, the two groups change over and those who were taking the placebo are given the active treatment, while those who were taking the active treatment receive the placebo. The result of this study gives a better idea of the effectiveness of the tested treatment.

DNA – Deoxyribonucleic acid. This is a long string of chemicals, like a complicated step-ladder, containing all the genetic information necessary for the production of another organism similar to the original.

Double-blind study – a study in which neither the investigator, nor the patient knows whether the patient is receiving active treatment or just a placebo. This ensures that the results are as independent as possible. A third party checks the results.

Hormone – a chemical messenger compound, produced and released into the bloodstream by endocrine organs (glands). Examples of hormones are: insulin, DHEA, GH, oestrogen, progesterone, testosterone, pregnenolone, melatonin.

Molecule – a chemical structure with individual chemical properties. Examples of molecules are proteins, DNA, enzymes, free radicals, sugars, aldehydes etc.

Pituitary gland – a small gland secreting several hormones, located on the midline towards the base of the brain.

Platelets – blood constituents which take part in the clotting of the blood. A high activity of platelets causes increased clotting, whereas a low activity may result in haemorrhage.

Placebo – dummy treatment. A placebo-controlled study is one which compares the effects of some proper treatment against the effects of placebo

Pro-oxidants – substances which enhance oxidation.

Further Reading

Coenzyme Q10 Phenomenon, Dr S Sinatra, Keats Publishing, Connecticut, 1998

DHEA Breakthrough, S A Cherniske, Ballantine Books, New York, 1997

Grow Young with HGH, R Klatz, HarperCollins, New York, 1997 (For more information regarding secretagogue products see www.antiaginginfo.net/compare.htm)

Methyl Magic, Craig Cooney, Andrews McMeel Publishing, Kansas City, 1999

Stay Young, Longer – Naturally, Dr Marios Kyriazis, Vega, London, 2001

Useful Addresses

SUPPLIERS OF CARNOSINE

In the USA and other parts of the world:– International Anti-aging Systems (including the Far East), Life Extension Foundation, Vitamin Research Products (for addresses, see below).

In the UK:– The Nutricentre, 7 Park Crescent, London W1N 3HE, tel.: 020 7436 5122, www.nutricentre.co.uk

In Australia:– www.betaalistine.com.au

Also from:
www.smart-drugs.com
www.integratedhealth.com

ORGANISATIONS

The British Longevity Society:– This is a UK based organisation which aims to inform the general public about the latest news in the field of anti-ageing medicine. It is where I can be contacted.
P.O. Box 71, Hemel Hempstead, HP3 9DN United Kingdom
www.antiageing.freeserve.co.uk
email: kyriazis@antiageing.freeserve.co.uk

Vespro Ltd:– The suppliers of the Free Radical Kit

www.vespro-europe.co.uk,

www.vesproeurope.com,

www.vespro.com

International Anti-Aging Systems (IAS):– IAS are a global organisation, the sponsors and organisers of the Monte Carlo Anti-Aging Conference. They publish regular bulletins and catalogues/directories, but they are unable to deliver to UK addresses.

Les Autelets, Sark GY9 0SF, Channel Islands, UK

tel.: 01144 8701514144

www.antiaging-systems.com

The Life Extension Foundation:– Members receive a monthly magazine with the latest information on all aspects of ageing. The Foundation also offers many other resources and products.

P.O. Box 229120, Hollywood, Florida 33022-9120, USA

www.lef.org

VRP (Vitamin Research Products):– They are a US-based company offering a variety of products, including carnosine.

3579 Hwy 50 East, Carson City, Nevada 89701 USA

tel.: 800 877 2447

www.vrp.com

email: mail@vrp.com

World Wide Health Corporation:– They can supply products and anti-ageing information.

WWH, Alderney GY1 5SS, UK

www.wwh-corp.com

American Academy of Anti-aging Medicine:– Some academics do not recognize this as an official organisation, but it does organize an annual conference on anti-ageing. It issues the *International Journal of Anti-Aging Medicine*, and other related publications. It runs an accreditation program for qualifications in anti-aging medicine, and has a record of practitioners from around the world.

1341 W Fullerton, Suite 111, Chicago IL 60614, USA

tel.: 773 528 43330

www.worldhealth.net

Index